WHERE TO BE BORN?

The debate and the evidence

Rona Campbell

Alison Macfarlane

Second edition

National Perinatal Epidemiology Unit
Oxford

At the time this second edition was being prepared Rona Campbell was a lecturer in the Department of Sociology and Social Policy at the Queen's University of Belfast. She is now an Honorary Research Fellow in the Division of Community Health of the United Medical and Dental Schools of Guy's and St. Thomas's Hospitals, University of London, based at the South East Institute of Public Health in Tunbridge Wells. Alison Macfarlane is Medical Statistician at the National Perinatal Epidemiology Unit. The first edition of this review arose out of work done while Rona Campbell was a PhD student at the London School of Hygiene and Tropical Medicine. Her project there was a survey of all births at home in England and Wales in 1979. This was done in association with the National Perinatal Epidemiology Unit and the Office of Population Censuses and Surveys. This second edition updates the first in the light of subsequent developments.

Published by
National Perinatal Epidemiology Unit
Radcliffe Infirmary
Oxford OX2 6HE

Cover design: Claire Montell
Printed by: Oxuniprint, Oxford University Press, Walton
                     Street, Oxford OX2 6DP
Trade distribution: Turnaround, 27 Horsell Road, London N5 1XL

Foreword to the Second Edition

Our main aim in this second edition has been to update the evidence on place of birth and to review the debate on policy which has taken place since the first edition was published in 1987.

The book retains its original format and starts by describing the way policies developed from the late nineteenth century up to the early 1980s. Next comes our review of the evidence. This opens with a new section outlining the methods and measures used in research and the merits and disadvantages of the various approaches taken. As the debate has moved on since 1987 and rather different policies have emerged, we have added a new closing section which comments on recent developments and the ways in which evidence has been brought into the debate.

In the foreword to our first edition we commented that because the debate focused on the place of birth rather than on the people who gave care at birth, it made midwives almost invisible. Since we wrote this, midwife-led care has re-emerged. It has taken a variety of forms and in some places has led to the designation of midwife-led units. Many schemes are still being evaluated but a few evaluations have already been published. A new section on midwifery care discusses these schemes and the increasing contribution made by midwives to research.

The first few years of this decade are witnessing huge changes within the health service. It is too early to assess the precise impact of these on maternity care. It is already obvious that costs of care are an important consideration even though evidence on the relative costs of giving birth in different places is fairly sparse. The work which has been done is reviewed in this edition. Rather more research has been undertaken on parents' views on place of birth and choice is also high on the political agenda. A section in this edition assesses the research published since 1987, along with some of the difficulties in obtaining and interpreting the views of people who use the services.

The upsurge of interest in the subject of where to be born is not peculiar to the United Kingdom. Increased interest in other countries has also led to the publication of new research. Nevertheless, as with the first edition, this review concentrates on evidence about different settings for birth in the United Kingdom.

Rona Campbell
Alison Macfarlane
June 1994

Foreword to the First Edition

This review is written primarily for the staff and users of the National Health Service in the United Kingdom. Although we have discussed some of the research done in other countries, we have made no attempt to be comprehensive.

This is because patterns of maternity care differ widely from country to country. For example, a general practitioner birth in Canada where, at the time of writing, there are no licensed midwives is likely to be different from one in the United Kingdom, where midwives play a major role. Similarly, the context and back up facilities for home births in the United Kingdom are very different from those in the Netherlands, which in turn differ from those in the United States.

We are also conscious that in focusing on the place of birth we may seem to have ignored the question of who provides the care. This reflects the fact that statistics have been compiled and the research work has been done in a way which tends to make midwives invisible. While they always have and still do attend the majority of births, past arguments have often centred on the position of GPs and obstetricians without taking into account the contribution of midwives and other staff. We are encouraged by the increasing tendency for midwives to do their own research and hope this will result in fuller information emerging in the future.

Rona Campbell
Alison Macfarlane
April 1987

Acknowledgments

We are grateful to Susan Walters for preparing the final manuscript for publication and to Suzanne Williams, Lyn Pilcher, Kay Pennick, Valerie Philcox, Rochelle Seifas and Frances Gifford who helped in other ways. We should also like to thank Miranda Mugford for permission to quote extensively from an article on costs of maternity care and other staff of the National Perinatal Epidemiology Unit who gave helpful advice, as did Iain Chalmers, Susan Williams, Irvine Loudon, Charles Webster and Eugene Declerq. Alison Macfarlane is funded by the Department of Health.

Figure 10 is reproduced by permission of *The Lancet* and Table 9 by permission of Marjorie Tew.

Contents

Introduction

Midwifery is an unusually emotive subject so, a priori, a very high
standard of statistical analysis or experimental approach would not
be expected.[1]

Archie Cochrane, *Effectiveness and efficiency*, 1972.

Controversies about where women should have their babies and
who should attend them in labour and at delivery have been raging
for at least two centuries.[2,3] Despite the extent to which some of
the protagonists have quoted statistics in support of their views, the
debate has always been hampered by the absence of reliable
statistical and epidemiological information. As Florence
Nightingale put it in her *Notes on lying-in institutions*:

It must be admitted, at the very outset of this enquiry that
midwifery statistics are in an unsatisfactory condition . . . but as
will afterwards be shown, with all their defects, midwifery statistics
point to one truth; namely, that there is a large amount of
preventable mortality in midwifery practice, and that, as a general
rule the mortality is far, far greater in lying-in hospitals than
among women lying-in at home.[4]

This book discusses the development of policies about giving birth
in different settings and reviews evidence about the risks and
benefits. The first edition, published in 1987, grew out of the
literature review for Rona Campbell's doctoral thesis on home
births in England and Wales in 1979.[5] It was thus started before
computerised databases were widely available and was therefore
based on a thorough manual search of relevant journals. Further
studies were added to the list as they emerged. While writing this

second edition the databases available through MEDLINE[6] and Bath University Interactive Data Services (BIDS)[7] have been searched to look for any publications which may have been missed.

This review is limited, quite deliberately, to studies comparing birth in different settings in the United Kingdom, except where there has been no relevant research from these islands. In some of these cases, selected studies from abroad are discussed to illustrate how the questions have been approached elsewhere. This choice to focus on settings within a single health care system is quite intentional. The circumstances of home and hospital birth and the roles played by different professions as birth attendants vary from country to country, so the conclusions from one country do not necessarily apply elsewhere. Comparisons between countries pose different questions which need to be considered separately.

Monitoring the debate about policy is by its very nature less amenable to systematic methods, given that the debate is not restricted to clinical and academic journals. It is conducted in many other places, including the media, parliament and encounters at both individual and organisational levels between clinicians, NHS managers and users of the services. The description of the policy debate given here relies largely on critical reading of official documents and parliamentary reports. While these present a partial view, they both reflect and influence statements and articles elsewhere.

While maternity care has changed beyond all recognition since Florence Nightingale's book was published in 1871, the statistics still fall short of what is needed. Despite this, much can be learned from them. As Florence Nightingale wrote,

Our only resource at present is to deal with such statistical information as we possess and to ascertain fairly what it tells us . . . [4]

To set the scene, we start by charting the change from home to institutional birth which has taken place during this century and the debate which accompanied it. We then go on to review the available research on the subject of the place of birth in the United Kingdom. In doing so, we suggest some conclusions which can be drawn from it, while pointing to the gaps and deficiencies in the evidence and questions which remain unanswered. This is followed by a new section discussing how evidence has been used in the debate since the first edition of *Where to be born?* was published in 1987.

The Debate

The move from home to institutional birth

Florence Nightingale was one of the many people who pointed to the raised mortality in the charitable lying-in hospitals during the nineteenth century and, indeed, in the preceding century when many of them were founded.[8,9] In the *Annual report of the Registrar General for the year 1841*, William Farr included a report on puerperal fever from Robert Storrs, a surgeon of Doncaster, and discussed other reports about puerperal fever in lying-in hospitals, commenting that 'the extent to which these institutions increase the danger of childbirth is now well known.'[10]

Over twenty years later, the *Pall Mall Gazette* carried a report of a survey of maternal deaths in the lying-in wards of 39 metropolitan workhouses in 1865. The death rate of 6.0 per thousand 'cases of childbirth' was higher than the 3.5 per thousand of the outdoor midwifery department of St George's Hospital. It was, however, lower than those of 'indoor establishments' run by charities, notably Queen Charlotte's Hospital 'which possesses a great reputation as a school of obstetric practice' where the mortality rate was 40.0 per thousand.[11]

At this time, however, most women delivered at home. The Select Committee on Midwives' Registration reported that in 1890, one per cent of births took place in workhouse infirmaries and 0.3 per cent in voluntary hospitals, most of which were the lying-in hospitals referred to above.[12] According to the results of a special survey published in 1909 in the *Minority report of the Poor Law Commission*, an estimated 1.2 per cent of births in England and Wales took place in workhouse infirmaries.[13] At this period, these births were all to women on poor relief. Since the passing of the 1834 Poor Law Amendment Act, local relieving officers had been responsible for deciding whether women in these circumstances should deliver in the local workhouse or at home with a midwife paid out of the poor rates. The choices were made largely in terms of cost to the ratepayers.

Maternity and child welfare schemes

The early years of this century were a time of public concern about infant mortality, and the Government was under political pressure to set up schemes for maternity and child welfare. This led to the 1907 Notification of Births Act which, as well as requiring the birth attendant to notify births, gave the Local Government Board powers to give grants to local authorities and voluntary societies for providing care for women and children. These powers were extended under the Notification of Births (Extension) Act of 1915.

Schemes included staff for home visiting of expectant mothers and babies, home helps, maternity centres with antenatal and infant welfare clinics and the provision of in-patient beds. A memorandum on the subject issued in 1915 by Arthur Newsholme, the Local Government Board's Chief Medical Officer, contained the following guidance on the 'provision of medical assistance at confinements':

The local authority may provide beds for patients suffering from complications arising during pregnancy or childbirth. These beds can be provided directly by the authority or by arrangement between them and an existing hospital. The necessity for reserving hospital beds for the treatment of puerperal fever and allied conditions must be borne in mind.

A local authority is also empowered, with the Board's consent to pay, in whole or in part, the fees for the doctor or midwife attending the confinement at home of necessitous women, and one half of such approved expenditure is paid by the Local Government Board.[14]

The Board phrased its views about hospital provision more positively in 1917 in a report on maternity and child welfare:

A complete scheme for maternity and child welfare should provide for hospital accommodation for complicated cases of pregnancy, for complications arising from parturition, such as puerperal fever in the mother or ophthalmia neonatorum in the child and for children found at the centres to be in need of treatment.[15]

Twilight sleep

A factor which played a major part in the move from home to hospital birth in North America was 'twilight sleep', a form of heavy sedation devised in Germany. It was mentioned briefly in the Local Government Board's report for 1918-19:

Twilight Sleep - increasing attention has been drawn during the year to the falling birth-rate and any proposals which may influence it must necessarily concern the Board. Among these is a method of conducting a confinement so that all recollection of its incidents is lost, there being apparently no record in the memory of their occurrence. This is known as the 'scopolamine morphine narcosis' or in popular terms 'twilight sleep'.[16]

Results of observations by the Section of Obstetrics and Gynaecology of the Royal Society of Medicine led to the conclusion that twilight sleep:

. . . could not be carried out at the patient's home, except for persons to whom the cost was immaterial. It would therefore seem that the wider adoption of this treatment must for the present be limited to hospitals. Such hospitals would require greatly increased nursing staff and a resident medical attendant, if they undertook the treatment.[16]

Although some people took up the idea of twilight sleep and it was used in general practice, it did not gain widespread use in this country. Its popularity had probably waned by the time that a campaign for pain relief had developed. This was spearheaded by the National Birthday Trust Fund, a voluntary organisation which was founded in 1928,[17,18] to improve maternity services for working class women.

Maternity homes

The idea of institutional delivery for women without complications had already emerged in the nineteenth century, but different sorts of institutions were envisaged.[4,19] In his Milroy lectures on *Deaths in childbed, a preventable mortality* given to the Royal College of Physicians in 1904,[20] William Williams reminded his audience of Florence Nightingale's observations on 'Military lying-in management' over thirty years earlier, when she suggested that:

Ordinary women have no need of long nursing after lying-in; it is all over in a few days after retirement and delivery in a rude compartment of a hut.[4]

Florence Nightingale had described two such huts at military camps, saying of one:

This hut does not form part of a hospital. It is a separate establishment solely for lying-in women as such accommodation should always be.[4]

It is clear that Williams did not envisage that such institutions should be hospitals. He plagiarised the caustic comments William Farr had made on lying-in hospitals over thirty years before, in the *Registrar General's report for 1870*:

Seeing how destitute of comforts, means and medical appliances many women are, the thought occurred to some benevolent person that they might be received and delivered in hospitals. It was the extension of the hospital system to midwifery cases, which have some analogy with wounds and injuries for which hospitals have been used from the date of their foundation. Contrary to expectations the advantages these institutions offered were over-balanced by one dread drawback; the mortality of mothers was not diminished; nay it became in some instances excessive; in other instances appalling.[21]

Williams also quoted William Farr's response to Florence Nightingale in the same report. There, Farr had coined the word 'natuary' for a place to which women without obstetric problems could retire to give birth:

When we consider the want of adequate accommodation in large towns for the wives of working men it must be evident that a certain number of them would find great comfort in being able to retire, as the soldier's wife does, into a hut for a few days until their trouble is over and for this surely arrangements might be made to enable them to pay beforehand by instalments. The natuary, clean and ventilated, armed with proper appliances and a midwife on the spot, would be more use than the mortuary.[21]

Similar arguments were advanced by the Local Government Board in its *Annual report for 1917-1918:*

The cessation of building and the over crowding of towns caused by the War have emphasized the need for maternity homes for women who cannot safely or conveniently be confined in their own homes. This need is being met by local authorities and by nursing associations and other voluntary agencies. These homes are usually established in existing houses adapted for this purpose. They are usually placed in charge of a matron who is a trained midwife and arrangements are made for the attendance of a doctor in emergencies. Many of these homes take complicated as well as normal cases.[22]

It was recommended that these homes should be built on the outskirts of towns and have gardens. The emphasis was not on 'safety' in the modern clinical sense but in providing both women and staff with a setting which offered better circumstances than most people's homes at this time.

With the passing in 1919 of the Ministry of Health Act, the Medical Department of the Local Government Board was absorbed into the new Ministry of Health. A division of Maternity and Child Welfare was set up with Dr Janet Campbell, in charge 'assisted by a staff of women doctors, nurses and midwives'.[23] The Welsh and Scottish Boards of Health, set up in the same year, took on responsibility for maternity and child welfare schemes in their countries.

Early in 1920 the Ministry of Health issued a *Memorandum in regard to maternity hospitals and homes*,[24] commenting in its annual report that:

> During the past year, 50 new maternity homes with over 500 beds have been provided by local authorities and voluntary agencies. Schemes for 20 other homes with a total of 250 beds are under consideration.[23]

The memorandum contained plans drawn by the Ministry of Health's architects for buildings of different sizes, ranging from a maternity home with 8 beds to a 120 bed hospital with four 30 bed pavilions, together with notes on their design. Introducing these, the Ministry explained the difference between homes and hospitals while acknowledging that they 'differ in degree rather than kind'. Both were intended to provide out-patient care and clinics and 'under proper conditions' give training for pupil midwives and medical students. The distinction was that:

> Maternity homes having up to 18 or 20 beds, should provide mainly for normal cases, miscarriages or cases of minor difficulty.[24]

On the other hand,

> ... maternity hospitals having 25 to 50 or an even greater number of beds are mainly required in the large towns ... They should be fully equipped for the treatment of all complications and disorders of pregnancy and labour, and for purposes of clinical treatment.

They should provide, primarily, for abnormal or difficult cases, but also for a certain number of straightforward confinements.[24]

As Figure 1 shows, the numbers of beds in municipal and voluntary homes increased steadily from 1915 onwards, although many were in converted buildings. In the first of a series of major reports on maternal mortality, published in 1924, Janet Campbell remarked that the Ministry's policy of setting up these homes for women without complications had been criticised on the grounds that:

> . . . the science and art of obstetrics would be far better served by the establishment of a few large, well equipped hospitals, with full facilities for teaching as well as treatment.[25]

She may have been referring to views similar to those expressed by Victor Bonney some five years previously in an address to the Obstetric Section of the Royal Society of Medicine. In putting the case for *Midwifery as a surgical art*, he said:

> Pregnancy is a state induced by the growth of a neoplasm; labour is a process accompanied by self-inflicted wounds, and the puerperium is the period of their healing. Midwifery concerns itself with the treatment of these three and is a pure surgical art, for the diseases of the newborn child are the province of the physician.[26]

He did not encourage intervention, however, as:

> Every manipulation within the birth canal, even the single examination to determine the position of the presenting part, carries with it a definite risk of conveying sepsis, which must be balanced against the advantages of the interference.[26]

Janet Campbell reiterated her position in a further report *The protection of motherhood*[27] published in 1927:

> It is not necessary to take the extreme view that all confinements should be regarded as surgical operations, and, therefore treated

in hospitals, to realise that sufficient beds to provide at least for abnormal and complicated cases, for patients living under such unsatisfactory conditions that they cannot safely be confined at home, for patients requiring antenatal observation and for septic cases - including abortions, are an essential part of a maternity service.[27]

The rise of the maternity hospital

As grants under the Maternity and Child Welfare Act were available for homes but not hospitals, statistics about the latter did not appear in the Ministry's reports in the 1920s and thus do not feature in Figure 1. Under the 1929 Local Government Act, the directly elected Poor Law Boards of Guardians were abolished and responsibility for Poor Law institutions including their infirmaries passed to local authorities. Many authorities expanded their infirmaries, including in many cases their maternity departments, and opened them to paying patients.[28] As Figure 1 shows, the numbers of beds rose considerably during the 1930s both in homes and hospitals, but the backbone of the service was still provided at home by domiciliary midwives employed by local authorities.[29]

In 1927, when the General Register Office first tabulated live births in England and Wales by place of delivery, 15 per cent of them took place in institutions, a category which included hospitals, nursing homes, maternity homes and Poor Law institutions.[30] The percentage of live births in institutions rose to 24 per cent in 1932[31] and 34.8 per cent in 1937.[32] Of the women sampled in the national survey of one week's births in 1946, 53.7 delivered in institutions.[33]

During the 1950s, the percentage of births taking place in hospital remained fairly static at around 65 per cent, before it rose steadily in the 1960s and 1970s.[34] As Figure 2 shows, this coincided with a fall in the total numbers of births. The percentage of births taking place outside the NHS in private and military hospitals decreased from 4.5 per cent in 1954 to 2.9 per cent in 1964 and 1.7 per cent in 1974, mainly reflecting the decreasing numbers of small private hospitals. In 1992, 96.5 per cent of all women delivering did so in NHS hospitals with consultant obstetric units, while only 1.4 per cent delivered in isolated general practitioner units, 0.7 per cent delivered in hospitals outside the NHS and 1.3 per cent delivered at home.[35]

In the 1920s and 1930s, the pressure for institutional care came from a variety of sources.[36] The Women's Co-operative Guild stressed the unsuitability of most working class women's homes for childbirth and their need for ten day's rest in hospital afterwards. Obstetricians, on the other hand, were more inclined to emphasise clinical factors. Middle class women campaigned for more maternity beds in hospitals where anaesthesia was becoming available.[37]

Yet, despite concern about maternal mortality, childbirth was still seen as essentially normal, as the British Medical Association put it in 1936,

> . . . a natural physiological event, though it is one involving complex, delicate and important processes. Departures from the normal occur in a small proportion of cases.[38]

Over the years, a variety of factors have contributed to change this approach to maternity care with an increasing tendency to see pregnancy and childbirth as hazardous processes in which medical assistance and intervention are often required[39,40,41] but in a statement to the press in 1936, the official view of the British Medical Association was still that:

> . . . all the available evidence demonstrates that normal confinements, and those which show only a minor departure from normal, can be more safely conducted at home than in hospital.[38]

In the same year, this view was supported by the British (later to become Royal) College of Obstetricians and Gynaecologists which, in a memorandum on a national maternity service, stated that:

> . . . adequate hospital provision for all cases could only be made at great expense: the results of domiciliary midwifery do not warrant such expenditure.[42]

Figure 1

Numbers of maternity beds, England and Wales, 1915-1992

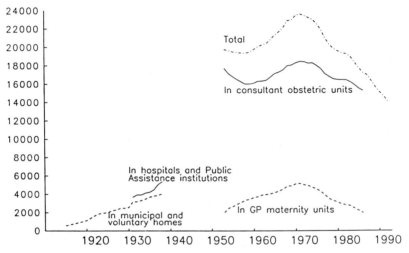

Source: Ministry of Health, DHSS, DH and Welsh Office

Figure 2

Births in institutions, England and Wales, 1920-1992

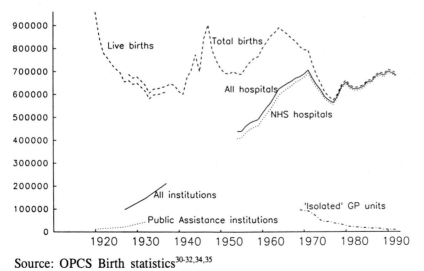

Source: OPCS Birth statistics[30-32,34,35]

Despite their agreement on this, the 1930s saw competition between obstetricians and GPs about who should be responsible for maternity care, much of which was actually provided by midwives.[29]

The tide was already turning, however. The *Registrar General's statistical review for 1932*, published in 1935, commented:

> The great increase which has taken place in the numbers of those seeking institutional treatment is due in part to increases in the facilities for such treatment, but is also assignable to changes, both economic and sentimental in the outlook of expectant mothers.[31]

Other changes were on the way, notably in the outlook for women who contracted puerperal sepsis, which we describe in some detail later.

It is perhaps in reaction to these changes that only a few years later in 1944, the Royal College of Obstetricians and Gynaecologists (RCOG) recommended maternity accommodation should be provided to allow for 70 per cent of all births to take place in hospital.[43] Ten years later, it called for all births to take place in hospital[44] and started to plan research, which it hoped would show this to be the safest policy.[45] Meanwhile the Second World War had an impact on maternity services. The Emergency Medical Services set up maternity homes in buildings such as church halls, offices and sometimes hospital premises to provide care for women who were temporarily evacuated from the most heavily bombed urban areas.[46]

The RCOG was involved in the birth survey which the National Birthday Trust Fund eventually undertook in 1958. As the Fund's Chairman Lady Juliet Rhys Williams put it in a private letter, written in July 1954, to the Prime Minister, Harold Macmillan:

> The Trust is at present financing a nation-wide statistical enquiry under the control of Professor Nixon of University College Hospital, with Ministry of Health approval, to discover whether there is any evidence - or otherwise - that the mothers and babies are, in fact safer in hospital than in their own homes. The pilot survey shows that they are, but it is not an easy thing to establish. If, as seems possible, the results are strikingly in favour of the

hospital, the Royal College of Obstetricians is likely to take the matter up in a big way, as they are anxious to support 100 per cent hospitalisation.[47]

Lady Juliet went on to propose a scheme involving more maternity homes, rather than increasing the numbers of places in consultant units. When the findings of the 1958 survey were published, they showed that mortality rates for births booked and delivered at home were not high compared with hospital births.[48] The Cranbrook Committee, which had been set up in April 1956 to review policies for the organisation of maternity services, published its report in 1959. In its paragraph 329 it recommended that:

. . . sufficient hospital maternity beds to provide for a national average of 70 per cent of all confinements to take place in hospital should be adequate to meet the needs of all women in whose case the balance of advantage appears to favour confinement in hospital.[49]

Hospital delivery was also becoming more popular with women, particularly after the National Health Service started. When the Association for Improvements in the Maternity Services was founded in 1960, it started to campaign for more hospital beds. Thus the selection of women to deliver in hospital was a recurring theme in Ministry of Health Annual Reports in the 1950s and 1960s when, in some parts of the country at least, demand outstripped supply. After consulting the Standing Advisory Committee on Maternity and Midwifery, the Ministry issued guidance in 1951 to hospital boards and local health authorities in its *Circular RHB(51)74*. This suggested that:

. . . priority should be accorded to all cases in which there are medical and obstetrical reasons for hospital care and where there are adverse social conditions, including bad housing. The first group would contain a high proportion of women having their first babies and those who already had four or more. It is most important that the assessment of social factors should be made by those most familiar with them - consequently the Medical Officer of Health is best placed to advise on the order of priority in the light of reports from his midwives and health visitors.[50]

A relatively long length of stay was recommended:

It is considered essential that patients admitted for confinement should be retained for a sufficient period - ten days is regarded as a minimum unless there are exceptional reasons why the patient may be discharged earlier to her home where the accommodation is good and attendance is known to be available.[50]

Later in the 1950s the emphasis shifted away from specific social needs and towards demographic factors, notably age and parity, as criteria for hospital delivery.

The target level of 70 per cent of deliveries taking place in institutions was achieved in 1964 and by 1968 the percentage of deliveries had risen to 80.6. The numbers of maternity beds in England and Wales increased by only 15 per cent between 1955 and 1968 while the total number of births increased by 18 per cent. This rise in the institutional delivery rate was therefore achieved by a reduction in the average length of stay. The average length of combined antenatal and postnatal stay declined from 12.1 days in 1955 to 8.0 days in 1968 for consultant beds, and from 11.1 to 6.8 days for GP beds[51]. Much of the decline in the length of postnatal stay in maternity beds preceded publication of the results of a number of experiments with schemes involving early discharge from hospital.[52-55]

As well as the decline in the length of stay in hospital there was a substantial fall over this period in the ratio of consultant staffed maternity beds to GP staffed maternity beds. In 1955 the ratio was 6.3 consultant beds to each GP bed but by 1968 this ratio had fallen to 3.7.[51] Meanwhile, as Figure 3 shows, the numbers of consultants in obstetrics and gynaecology, which had been increasing steadily since the NHS started, rose more steeply in the 1960s. In addition, the numbers of local authority midwives working in the community decreased, while the numbers of hospital midwives rose, as Figure 4 shows.

The trend since 1970 has been towards consultant care in large specialised units, just as Victor Bonney recommended in 1919.[26] This, taken together with the continuing and long standing emphasis on trying to identify problems during antenatal care and, more recently, the promotion of preconceptional care reflects changes in the way society and professionals view pregnancy and childbirth[39-41] not simply as natural events but rather as processes requiring medical supervision.

The changing role of general practitioners

The rise in the proportion of GP staffed beds coincided with the development of integrated general practitioner units where general practitioners and community midwives could carry out their obstetric and midwifery practice with the full facilities of the obstetric hospital at their disposal if required. Reports of this type of unit began to appear in the mid 1950s[56,57] and in 1959 the Cranbrook Report[49] recommended that all general practitioner obstetricians should have access to maternity beds within or adjacent to consultant maternity hospitals or general hospitals with a maternity department. Despite this, the development of integrated GP units was probably impeded by the legal restrictions which prevented domiciliary midwives, who were employed by local authorities, from working in places other than the mother's home. These restrictions were abolished under the Health Services and Public Health Act 1968[51]. From the 1974 reorganisation until 1991, all NHS midwives were employed by health authorities. Since April 1991 they have been employed by directly managed units and NHS trusts.

By the late 1950s, maternity homes, many of which had been established between the wars, had become known as 'isolated GP maternity units'. This change in name to 'GP unit' is symptomatic of a change in emphasis which occurred despite the fact that midwives were still responsible for supervising most of the deliveries. Units are described as 'isolated' if they are either freestanding units or are in a hospital without a consultant obstetric unit. The use of the word 'isolated' came to imply more than just

Figure 3

NHS consultants in obstetrics and gynaecology, England and Wales, 1950-1992

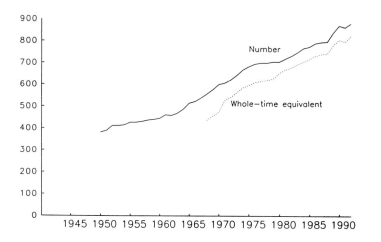

Source: Ministry of Health, DHSS, Welsh Office and NHS Executive

Figure 4

Whole time equivalent numbers of midwives, England and Wales, 1953-1987

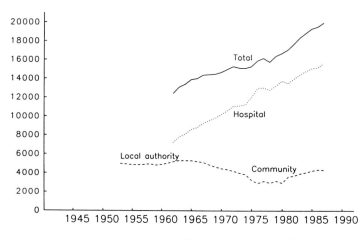

Source: Ministry of Health, DHSS and Welsh Office

geographic distance from consultant obstetric units. The term 'isolated' implied that such units were not part of modern mainstream maternity care. In its definition of a 'General practitioner unit' the report of the 1958 British Perinatal Mortality Survey noted that such units did not have resident medical officers, that anaesthetic facilities were limited and 'in general the facilities should be thought of as domiciliary obstetrics under good conditions rather than as an obstetric hospital.'[48]

A study in the Oxford area in 1962 documented dangers associated with booking high risk patients for delivery in 'isolated' general practitioner units, pointing specifically to the hazards associated with transfer of women during labour to specialist care.[58]

In 1970, when maternity policy was reviewed again in the Peel Report, only 12.4 per cent of deliveries occurred at home. The Peel Committee recognised the continuing trend towards universal hospitalisation and gave its official blessing to the policy when it recommended in its paragraph 248 that:

We consider that the greater safety of hospital confinement for mother and child justifies the objective of providing sufficient hospital facilities for every woman who desires or needs to have a hospital confinement. Even without specific policy direction the institutional confinement rate has risen from 64.4 per cent in 1957 to 80.7 per cent in 1968, and shows every sign of continuing to rise, so that discussion of the advantages and disadvantages of home or hospital confinement is in one sense academic.

The Peel Committee went on in paragraph 277 to say that:

We think that sufficient facilities should be provided to allow for 100 per cent hospital delivery. The greater safety of hospital confinement for mother and child justifies this objective.[51]

This was written at the end of a period when, as Figure 5 which is derived from the Peel Report shows, an increase in the number of maternity beds coincided with a dramatic fall in the fertility rate and in the numbers of births. Throughout the 1970s, further reports focused professional and public attention on the maternal

Figure 5

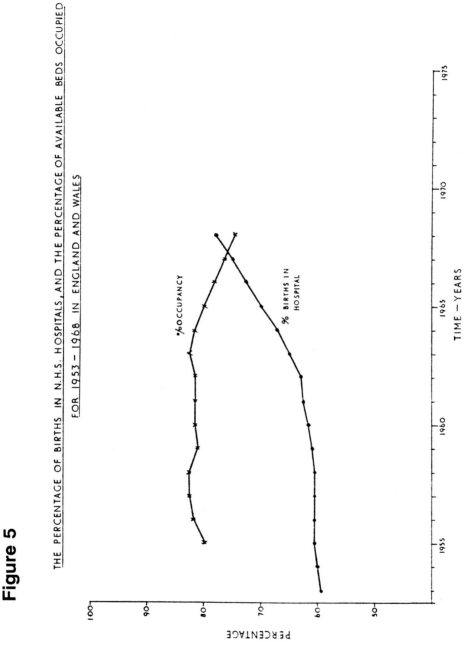

THE PERCENTAGE OF BIRTHS IN N.H.S. HOSPITALS, AND THE PERCENTAGE OF AVAILABLE BEDS OCCUPIED
FOR 1953 – 1968 IN ENGLAND AND WALES

Reproduced from the Peel Report on *Domiciliary midwifery and maternity bed needs*.[51]

and child health services and the emphasis shifted from mothers to babies. In 1971, the Sheldon Report claimed that 'evidence is quoted that modern intensive care not only would reduce perinatal mortality still further but also would reduce handicaps among surviving babies'.[59]

In 1976, the report of the Committee on Child Health Services[60] supported the proposals of the Peel and Sheldon Committees, while a DHSS policy document, *Priorities for health and personal social services in England* put the case for reducing levels of provision of maternity services in response to falling birth rates. It advised that:

. . . the best way of reducing provision to appropriate levels will need to be considered carefully in the light of all the existing facilities in each locality. . . . In some there may be grounds for reducing the level of provision in consultant units; in others a better course would be to make available the resources of general practitioner units to other services which need them urgently.[61]

In 1977, a second policy document, *The way forward*, pointed to regional and social class differences in perinatal mortality rates and stated that 'concentration of provision in properly equipped and staffed units is likely to lead to improved standards of care for the newborn'[62] and spoke of 'under-used and inefficient maternity units' being closed.[62]

The numbers of 'isolated' GP units fell from 226 in 1973 to 151 in 1978. The proportion of institutional births taking place in such units fell from 12.8 per cent to 5.7 per cent over the same period.[63] Meanwhile, it was estimated that the numbers of deliveries in the integrated type of GP unit rose from 6.1 per cent of all deliveries in 1970 to 9.1 per cent in 1975.[64] The culmination of these developments was the recommendation made by the House of Commons Social Services Committee in 1980 that:

An increasing number of mothers be delivered in large units; selection of patients is improved for small consultant units and isolated GP units; and that home delivery is phased out further.[63]

In accordance with a recommendation in the Committee's report, the government set up the Maternity Services Advisory Committee as a 'service oriented committee that is representative of all the interests in perinatal medicine'.[65] It made many suggestions for improving maternity care. On place of delivery, it said 'As unforeseen complications can occur in any birth, every mother should be encouraged to have her baby in a maternity unit where emergency facilities are readily available',[65] but did not specify in detail the complications or the facilities required to deal with them.

These recommendations echoed one made by the Cranbrook Committee 20 years earlier that:

> . . . a consultant obstetrician should have overall responsibility for the supervision of general practitioner maternity beds . . .

since, in the Committee's opinion:

> . . . the practice of obstetrics requires the exercise of special skill and experience and that there is not enough domiciliary maternity work available to enable every general practitioner to obtain and maintain the necessary standard of skill.[49]

During the past twenty five years, alterations in medical education have led to a reduction in the amount of obstetric experience that doctors have upon qualification. Furthermore, as long ago as 1970, the Peel Committee observed that:

> National figures show that domiciliary midwives are becoming less concerned with patients in labour and increasingly occupied with the postnatal nursing of patients discharged early from hospital. This change made it difficult to secure sufficient clinical experience for pupil midwives conducting cases on the district.[51]

This is even more true today and means that the proportion of midwives who have substantial experience of home delivery is continuously decreasing. The way the role of community midwives changed is illustrated in Figure 6 and the corresponding changes for general practitioners are shown in Figure 7. Changes since the late 1980s cannot be monitored through the statistical series shown in

Figure 6

The changing role of community midwives, England and Wales, 1949-87

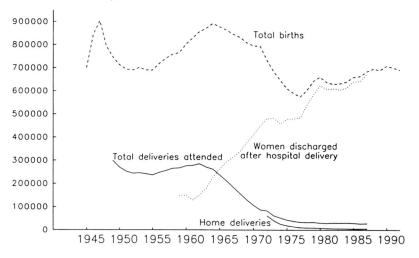

Source: Ministry of Health, DHSS and Welsh Office

Figure 7

Claims by GPs for fees for maternity care, England and Wales 1963-88

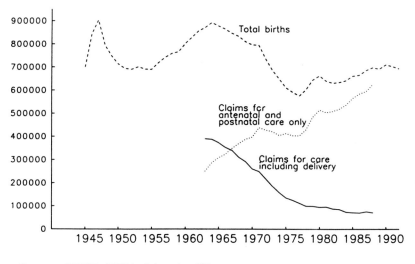

Source: DHSS, FP24 claims by GPs

Figures 6 and 7. After 1987, the only national data collected about the work of community midwives was the numbers of 'face-to-face' contacts they made, without any mention of their purpose. Since 1989, data about general practitioners' claims for fees for maternity care have been collected on a different basis from those shown in Figure 7 and are incompatible with them. It is also not possible to update Figure 4 as the Welsh Office no longer makes a distinction between nurses and midwives in its statistics. While this distinction is still made in England, it is increasingly unclear whether the subdivision into 'hospital' and 'community' is an adequate reflection of recent developments in midwifery.

As will be seen later, very little evidence was put forward by the various committees to support their recommendations for changes in the place of delivery, or as Archie Cochrane put it:

> . . . it is surprising how successive committees have been content to accept trends as something God-given which must be followed, instead of demanding a more rigorous analysis of causality.[1]

Nevertheless the changes have been implemented to a very large extent. This suggests either tacit agreement amongst the relevant professional groups that these changes were both necessary and efficacious,[66] or an absence of power on the part of those who disagreed with the changes to stop them.

Indeed, the story might have ended here, had not the prevailing orthodoxy been repeatedly challenged by Marjorie Tew, who has worked tirelessly, at her own expense, to analyse data about the place of delivery. Although we do not necessarily share all her conclusions, we should like to record our appreciation of the work she has done to present alternative analyses of the statistics, thereby keeping the issue alive. While at the forefront, Marjorie Tew was not alone in producing relevant analyses. The important work by John Ashford and other contributors to a book *The place of birth* edited by John Davis and Sheila Kitzinger should not be overlooked.[67]

The Evidence

The development of current policy on place of birth has rested on two fundamental assumptions. The first was that hospitals were the safest place for all women to give birth and the second was that the decline in perinatal and neonatal mortality was a consequence of the move from home to hospital birth. These assumptions were rarely, if ever, questioned. This section reviews evidence comparing birth in different settings. In doing so, it discusses whether the assumptions underlying the recommendation that all women should give birth in hospital, are justified, whether mortality should be regarded as the only measure of 'safety' and what other factors should be taken into account. The section opens by discussing how the evidence should be assessed, in terms of what is measured and what methods are used for making comparisons. These considerations determine which questions can and cannot be answered.

Assessing the evidence

WHAT SHOULD BE MEASURED?

Traditionally, mortality in women and babies has been used as a measure in comparing the safety of birth in different settings. Table 1 shows how the death rates commonly quoted are defined. For many years now, the numbers of women dying in pregnancy, childbirth or after the birth have been too low to form a basis for statistical comparisons, even though individual deaths are still audited through the Confidential Enquiry into Maternal Deaths.

Table 1

Definitions of stillbirth and infant mortality rates

Stillbirth rate $=$ $\dfrac{\text{Stillbirths x 1000}}{\text{Live births } + \text{ stillbirths}}$

Perinatal mortality rate $=$ $\dfrac{(\text{Stillbirths} + \text{deaths at 0-6 days after live birth}) \times 1000}{\text{Live births } + \text{ stillbirths}}$

Early neonatal mortality rate $=$ $\dfrac{\text{Deaths at 0-6 days after live birth x 1000}}{\text{Live births}}$

Late neonatal mortality rate $=$ $\dfrac{\text{Deaths at 7-27 days after live birth x 1000}}{\text{Live births}}$

Neonatal mortality rate $=$ $\dfrac{\text{Deaths at 0-27 days after live birth x 1000}}{\text{Live births}}$

Postneonatal mortality rate $=$ $\dfrac{\text{Deaths at 1-11 months after live birth x 1000}}{\text{Live births}}$

Infant mortality rate $=$ $\dfrac{\text{Deaths under the age of 1 year after live birth x 1000}}{\text{Live births}}$

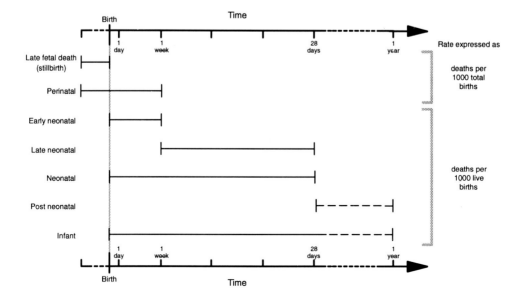

As maternal deaths became fewer, studies of place of delivery tended to focus on mortality in babies. In turn, with the increasing survival of very ill newborn babies past the first week of life, analyses tend to take into account deaths throughout the first month of life and use stillbirth and neonatal mortality rates.

In recent years, even stillbirth and neonatal mortality rates have fallen to a low level, particularly among women selected to have planned deliveries in low technology settings. This has two implications. Firstly, the numbers of adverse events are so small as to make statistical comparisons unreliable. In England and Wales in 1991, there were 3,254 stillbirths and 3,006 neonatal deaths in total but only 6 stillbirths and 17 neonatal deaths among babies born in isolated general practitioner units.[68] There were 63 stillbirths and 60 neonatal deaths among babies born at home. An unknown but probably small proportion of these births will have been planned to occur at home. Some of the stillbirths occurred before the onset of labour and are thus unlikely to be a consequence of the place of birth. Of the neonatal deaths among babies born at home, 28, that is nearly half, were known to have had birthweights under 1500g.

Secondly, the risk of death to mother or baby is now so small that women seeking low technology care may no longer perceive death as a major threat. The emphasis still placed on the need to reduce stillbirth and infant mortality rates means that they continue to be a concern for professionals, however. This is particularly so for those who began practice in an era when obstetric flying squads calls to women in difficult circumstances at home or in small maternity units were not uncommon.

Nevertheless, in choosing criteria for assessing the risks and benefits of different settings for birth, the emphasis is moving towards other measures, notably morbidity or health status, in terms of illness or disability, in women and babies. For healthy babies born at term, appropriate measures include infections, unexpected serious illness and problems in the neonatal period and Apgar scores, although the latter have been widely criticised. Health status later in childhood, in relation to circumstances at birth, has also become a concern, although this tends to be in the context of children who were born very small and ill and survive after intensive high technology care and hence may be less relevant to this document. For women, there is evidence of widespread morbidity in terms of problems in the postnatal period and later on.[69] A small number of studies have looked at these in relation to the place of delivery. In comparison with mortality, the choice of measures of morbidity is less clear cut, and there can be mismatches between women's and professionals' views of the relative importance of different types of morbidity. Morbidity is also less easy to measure and requires specific follow-up surveys.

With greater financial constraints on the health service, the perceived costs of different forms of care play an increasingly important role in decisions about the types of care which are provided. When comparing costs, it is important to take into account the costs of using the service as well as those of providing it. Furthermore, the way in which health care costs are met from different budgets can affect the preferred options of organisations providing care.

It is becoming acknowledged that parents' views about the care they receive are an important factor to consider when comparing birth in different settings. This may well interact both directly and indirectly with the morbidity women experience, as women's positive and negative reactions to the care they receive can affect their progress in labour.[70]

As a measurement of outcome, mortality has the advantage of relating to a defined event. Compared with mortality, both morbidity and parents' views are more difficult to assess and some important factors cannot easily be reduced to quantitative measures. If long term morbidity is to be considered, it follows that additional time is needed before conclusions can be drawn.

All these issues will play an increasingly important role in planning future work on delivery in different settings, but most past research used mortality as a criterion. It is therefore relevant to consider how mortality rates should be interpreted. This is because crude mortality rates, which are derived from total numbers of births and deaths without taking any other factors into account, can be misleading if they are used as simple indicators of the quality of midwifery, obstetric and paediatric care for a given place of delivery. It is therefore important to analyse the data in fuller detail.

Two major factors associated with stillbirths, perinatal and neonatal mortality are congenital malformations incompatible with life, and the pathology associated with low birthweight.[71] Congenital anomalies were given as a 'main fetal cause' for 7 per cent of stillbirths and 29 per cent of all neonatal deaths in England and Wales in 1991.[68] When neonatal deaths and stillbirths with congenital malformations mentioned on the certificate as a 'main fetal cause' were excluded, along with babies whose birthweights were missing, babies weighing under 2500g accounted for 58 per cent of stillbirths and 78 per cent of neonatal deaths of babies with known birthweight in England and Wales in 1991.[68]

A number of studies[72-74] have shown a high degree of association between low birthweight, socio-economic disadvantage and ethnic origin. Also Asian women and to a lesser extent women of Afro-Caribbean origin tend, on average, to have babies of lower birthweight than white women.[34,68,75] It is not clear to what extent this is a consequence of socio-economic disadvantage. Because these factors are an integral part of many women's earlier background and current circumstances, it is clear that crude mortality rates are not sensitive indicators of the quality of the maternity services. Furthermore, as these factors vary significantly throughout the country, appropriate methods should be used to take variations in them into account. There is no unanimity about which method is ideal, but there is general agreement that the use of crude statistics which do not take account of these factors is inappropriate.[76-80] In particular, high crude mortality rates in areas with disadvantaged populations may be largely a reflection of poor socio-economic conditions, although they may additionally reflect deficiencies which can exist in the care available to such populations.

Interpretation is further complicated by the way that the debate about place of delivery is often conducted as if it is simply a matter of two extremes, home or hospital.[81,82] In reality there exists a continuum of patterns of delivery care ranging from planned and unplanned birth outside hospital, at home or elsewhere, going to hospital for delivery only under a 'domino' scheme, delivery as an in-patient in an isolated or an integrated GP or midwife led maternity unit, or in a specialist consultant obstetric unit. Within a consultant obstetric unit, delivery may be supervised entirely by midwives, or may involve junior doctors with varying levels of experience, or a more experienced obstetrician.

Although choice of place of delivery may largely determine the pattern of antenatal and postnatal care, there may still be variation within the groups. For example, women delivering in a consultant obstetric unit may receive antenatal care based either in the consultant obstetric unit or in their GP's practice or both. In any of these settings, the role of midwives can vary from being the main caregiver to one of assisting doctors. This variety in the patterns of care makes evaluation yet more difficult. In addition, although the majority of deliveries are still conducted by midwives, the argument is often conducted in terms of the relative merits of GPs and obstetricians.[83]

There are also considerable differences between the staff within each profession in terms of their clinical skills and experience, their ability to work with others and their skills in communicating with parents. This may well be the crucial factor rather than the setting in which birth takes place, but it is not easily measurable and few studies have attempted to do so. A further problem besetting analyses of place of delivery is that women may not give birth in the place they originally intended. Their plans can change, either intentionally, for example from midwife to consultant care if complications arise, or unintentionally, for example from hospital to home birth if they go into labour unexpectedly and give birth quickly.

WHAT METHODS SHOULD BE USED?

The least biased way of making comparisons between similar groups of people receiving different forms of care is to do a randomised trial.[84] Despite this, most of the evidence available for us to review has been correlational, that is, based on observational data which have not been collected as part of studies with an experimental design. Even in the studies where attempts were made to control for the selection biases which confound place of delivery analyses, it is still difficult to assess the extent to which differences observed in outcomes are directly attributable to differences between places of birth.

George Bernard Shaw confessed to being out of his depth as far as the technique of correlation was concerned, but showed that he was only too aware of the dubious way in which it could be used when he wrote in his preface to *The doctor's dilemma*:

> To advertise any remedy or operation, you have only to pick out all the most reassuring advances made by civilization, and boldly present the two in relation of cause and effect: The public will swallow the fallacy without a wry face. It has no idea of the need for what is called a control experiment.[85]

A 'control experiment' or a randomised controlled trial is the only method by which it is possible to overcome fully the problem of selection biases and produce an unbiased assessment of the mortality and morbidity risks associated with the different places of birth. This type of experimental approach is now widely used to assess the efficacy of a wide range of obstetric, midwifery and neonatal practices.[86] Because the mortality rate associated with planned home delivery is so low, however, the numbers of participants needed in order to detect significant differences between the mortality in babies born to women delivering at different locations are now prohibitively high compared with the numbers of home births.[87]

In the 1960s or 1970s when substantially more women were giving birth at home, it would have been possible to do such an experiment. Unfortunately, this opportunity was missed by the successive committees who made recommendations about the place of delivery. This is because the issue at the time was meeting the demand for hospital delivery and selection of women for hospital birth when demand for places outstripped the supply. In addition, randomised trials were not yet widely used at this time.

It is certainly not too late to do randomised trials to answer other questions, however. In such studies, experimental methods can be useful to compare parents' views about, and the morbidity associated with the various places of delivery. This was done, for example, in a randomised trial comparing the use of a birthroom and a labour ward for delivery,[88] and in evaluating a 'home from home' scheme in Leicester[89].

Although the many strengths of randomised trials are widely recognised, they are not without problems.[90] The difficulty of organising trials to answer the types of question discussed in this book should not be underestimated. Because of the ways hypotheses have to be formulated, the questions to be answered may be relatively narrow and it is not always clear that the results can be generalised to other settings.

As a result, assessment of the safety of birth at home and in other low technology settings, has to rely on descriptive research in which it is virtually impossible to make comparative statements unless natural experiments occur. These are instances in which because of local circumstances, comparable groups of women receive different forms of care. For example, a study in Oxford compared women who booked to deliver in an integrated GP unit with similar women whose GPs were not involved in care during delivery.[91]

It is also possible to do case control studies, or non-randomised cohort studies in which attempts are made to match comparable women who have chosen different types of care but it is more difficult to avoid biases in this case. In particular, it is always a problem to decide how closely to try to match women, and whether doing so will obscure important comparisons. Another approach is to compare subsets of women separately. For example, it has been suggested that mortality rates should be calculated separately for birthweight groups after first excluding multiple births and lethal congenital malformations.[78] In each approach problems can arise if factors are aggregated to form 'risk prediction' scores. These are designed to predict rates for groups of people rather than adverse events in individuals. Even for groups, they tend to have a poor predictive value.[92,93]

As was mentioned above, these constraints make it different to draw conclusions which directly compare different settings for birth. Nevertheless, there is much information which can be derived from observational data which are still of considerable value provided that their limitations are borne in mind. This section continues by reviewing the considerable body of data about mortality, before going on to look at research on morbidity, costs of care and users' views.

Mortality and the place of birth

Interpreting changes over time

The Peel Committee's assumption about the nature of the relationship between mortality and the place of delivery was articulated more forcibly in 1984 by Alison Munro, chair of the Maternity Services Advisory Committee:

> The practice of delivering nearly all babies in hospital has contributed to the dramatic reduction in stillbirths and neonatal deaths and to the avoidance of many child handicaps.[65]

The same assumption was repeated by a Department of Health official when giving evidence to the House of Commons Health Committee in 1991. One of them said:

> We have some figures comparing 1955 when 33 per cent of babies were born at home, with 1989, . . . when less than 2 per cent were born at home. . . . When one-third of the babies were born at home in 1955 the perinatal mortality rate was at 37.4 per thousand still and live births, and it is now 8.3.[94]

Unlike its predecessor, the House of Commons Health Committee questioned the assumption that because these changes occurred at the same time, this established cause and effect.

A number of detailed analyses of the statistical association between the falls over time in both the perinatal mortality rate and the proportion of births at home[95-101] do not support the claims made above. Instead, they suggest that the relation is likely to be coincidental rather than causal.

One of these analyses used data from the Cardiff Births Survey[95] and showed that while the proportion of births occurring at home in the area covered by the survey fell from 1 in 5 in 1965 to 1 in 100 in 1973, the authors were unable to detect a decrease in the crude perinatal mortality rate, nor in death rates attributed to causes which were deemed preventable.   Another study used maternity records of women booked for delivery in hospitals with consultant obstetric facilities in Newcastle upon Tyne during the period 1960 to 1969. This analysis revealed similar patterns in the declines in perinatal mortality rates for home and institutional births.[96]

By 1981, the proportion of births in England and Wales taking place at home had fallen to 1.0 per cent, and it remained around this level throughout the 1980s, falling slightly to 0.9 per cent between 1985 and 1988, before a small but steady rise to 1.1 per cent in 1991 and 1.3 per cent in 1992.[35] In contrast with this static picture, perinatal mortality fell by 21 per cent from 11.8 per thousand total births in 1981 to 8.9 per thousand in 1987, and then fell by a further 15 per cent to 7.6 per thousand in 1992.[35] Figures 8 and 9 show how the decline in the perinatal mortality rate followed a different pattern to changes over time in the proportion of home births.

Marjorie Tew analysed changes in the percentages of births in hospital and in perinatal mortality rates in England and Wales as a whole and in each of the 15 hospital board regions over the period 1962-71. She found no statistical association between the year to year changes in mortality and the percentage of births in hospital.[97] In a later analysis covering the years 1969-78, she found a statistically significant negative association between falls in perinatal mortality and increases in the percentage of births in hospital.   In other words, above average annual increases in hospitalisation tended to be accompanied by below average falls in perinatal mortality.   She stated that 'this strongly supports the conclusion that increased hospitalisation adversely affected mortality.'[98]

Both this statement and those quoted earlier are equally unjustified as statistical association does not prove causation.   On the other hand, the lack of association found in Marjorie Tew's

Figure 8

Perinatal mortality England and Wales, 1964-92

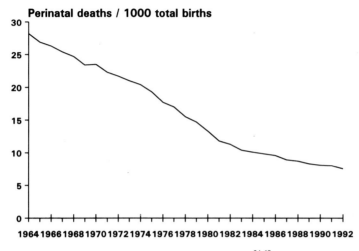

Source: OPCS Mortality statistics, Series DH3[34,68]

Figure 9

Percentage of deliveries at home, England and Wales, 1964-92

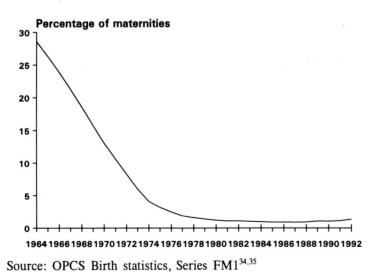

Source: OPCS Birth statistics, Series FM1[34,35]

analysis of data for 1962-71 suggests there was no causal relationship in this period.

The same is true of an analysis in which she found no statistical association between regional perinatal mortality rates and regional hospitalisation rates within each of the years 1963 to 1971.[97] It is interesting to note that, similarly, no association was observed in a study of regional perinatal mortality rates in the Netherlands in 1982.[99] Although only about two thirds of the births took place in hospital, there was considerable regional variation ranging from 50.3 per cent of births in Friesland to 74.2 per cent in Noord-Holland.

A study of the association between the combined stillbirth and neonatal mortality rates and hospital delivery rates between 1956 and 1969 in local authority areas of England and Wales[72] showed that in each year from 1956 to 1967, areas with above average hospital delivery rates tended to have below average mortality rates. The strength of this association weakened over time, however, and the position was reversed in 1968 and 1969. As the proportion of hospital deliveries increased even further between 1970 and 1973, the association with low mortality rates became even more tenuous.[100] Analyses subdivided by birthweight showed that throughout the entire period, higher hospital delivery rates tended to be associated with lower mortality rates in the group weighing less than 2501g. On the other hand, in babies weighing over 2500g, high mortality rates tended to be associated with high hospital delivery rates from 1964 onwards.[72,100] More recently, over the years 1987-91, consistent rises in the admittedly low proportions of home births[35] in some regions were not accompanied by increases in mortality.[68]

Turning to differences between countries, the perinatal mortality rates in Denmark and the Netherlands were compared over a period when home births were almost completely phased out in Denmark but not in the Netherlands. It was found, however, that the absolute levels of and trends in perinatal mortality rates for two countries were very similar.[101] International comparisons pose many problems, however. For example, there is considerable variation between countries in the way in which maternity services are organised. In particular, the role of midwives and the setting in which the midwives work in the Netherlands is different from that in the United Kingdom.[102] Comparisons are further frustrated by differences both in the regulations about birth and death registration and in the ways they are interpreted and applied.[34,103]

In addition, most of the analyses mentioned above rely on crude mortality statistics which do not allow for any of the other factors which can influence the outcome of pregnancy. The rest of this section discusses analyses which have attempted to do this.

Maternal mortality and the place of birth

Maternal deaths are now too rare to be used in current analyses. Although past maternal mortality rates were often uncorrelated with infant mortality rates,[104] it is relevant to look at the way maternal mortality data were handled. Not only is it of interest to see how the problems of measurement and interpretation were tackled, but more importantly how the results were influential in shaping current policies.

In the nineteenth century, as we have seen, hospitals were more dangerous than other places of birth.[2,3,5,8,10,11,22] Furthermore, Robert Rentoul, a doctor with an interest in having deliveries conducted by doctors in women's own homes, alleged that mortality rates in most charitable lying-in hospitals might have been even higher had they not excluded the very women who were at highest risk of either losing their baby or dying themselves. These were unmarried women, women pregnant for the first time and women with no child living.[105]

The high mortality in workhouse infirmaries was commonly attributed solely to the poor health and deprived condition of the women delivering there. The minority report of the Poor Law Commission challenged this in 1909, pointing as well to the inadequate care and unsavoury conditions in some infirmaries.[13]

Towards the end of the nineteenth century many lying-in hospitals attempted to adopt aseptic and antiseptic procedures to prevent mortality from sepsis. William Williams, in his Milroy lectures, presented data from Queen Charlotte's Hospital about deaths in the hospital from the time of its rebuilding in 1857 until 1902, and deaths of patients of the 'external department' delivering in their own homes. Hospital mortality rates reached a very much lower level from the mid 1880s on, compared with those earlier in the century. For women delivering at home, Williams commented,

> The mean rate for the period of 21 years was 1.7 which is extremely satisfactory and much lower than the rate in the internal department, but this is not to be wondered at when one remembers that the majority of the worst cases are brought into hospital care after labour commences and that a large number undergo some of the major operations.[20]

A major report on maternal mortality, published in 1916 by the Local Government Board, included an analysis by Isabella Cameron, who compared mortality rates for women delivering in four hospitals and two out-patient departments. The data were derived from their annual reports. She was hampered by:

> The paucity of available statistics under this heading and the lack of comparability of such statistics as are given, owing to different methods of compilation.[106]

Despite this, she found raised death rates in the hospitals and commented that:

> The larger death rate from eclampsia and from puerperal fever in maternity hospitals than in the general population is doubtless due to the fact that these cases are exceptionally difficult to deal with at home, and hospital treatment is largely sought for them. The various septic conditions grouped together as puerperal fever give rise to a considerable number of deaths in hospital practice.[106]

As we have seen earlier, the risk of maternal mortality did not loom large in the arguments for institutional birth after the First World War. Except for those women deemed to be 'complicated cases' the undesirability of many women's housing conditions was seen as the major criterion. Indeed the focus was on the risks of puerperal sepsis from which reported death rates were often higher in hospital, possibly for the reasons identified above.

In a Ministry of Health report published in 1932 on *High maternal mortality in certain areas*, Janet Campbell, Isabella Cameron and Dilys Jones commented that:

> Criticisms are not seldom made of the high maternal death rate which occurs in maternity hospitals. This is explained partly by the fact that the proportion of difficult cases is large, and also by the reception of emergency cases, many of them actually moribund on admission.[107]

A review of maternal mortality at Queen Charlotte's Hospital confirmed this.[108]

This point was reiterated by Munro Kerr and Hector MacLennan in a report on maternal mortality in Glasgow Royal Maternity Hospital from 1926-30:

> To concentrate more particularly on the institutional problem we venture to suggest that the following additional factors play an important part:
> (a) Type of case admitted;
> (b) Nature of the population served by the institution;
> (c) Organisation of the institution.

> The mortality and morbidity rate of institutions such as our own which admit any type of emergency as, for example, the 'failed forceps' and the 'incomplete abortion' will naturally be relatively higher than that in institutions which deal almost exclusively with the booked case.[109]

They stressed this point by noting that the Ministry of Health's *Interim report on maternal mortality*[110] 'in quoting the excellence of results in certain institutions fail to specify the type of case admitted.'[109]

Whatever the record of individual institutions, it is clear that over the years 1915 to 1935, when the proportion of women delivering in them rose, the maternal mortality rate did not fall. If anything

Figure 10

Maternal mortality, England and Wales, 1847-1992

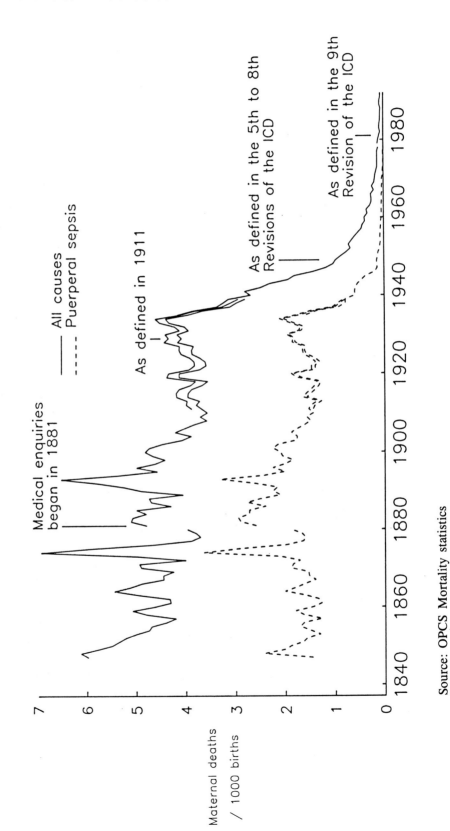

Source: OPCS Mortality statistics

it rose slightly, as Figure 10 shows, and the increase was in deaths attributed to puerperal sepsis.

The Ministry's *Interim report* commented on the improved outlook for 'abnormal cases' when delivering in a hospital with facilities for dealing with severe haemorrhage, eclampsia and operative or difficult delivery. On the other hand, it pointed to the greater risk of death from sepsis and pointed out that 47.7 per cent of the deaths from sepsis which it had studied, followed normal labour.[110]

It would appear, although there are no national statistics to verify it, that the move towards institutional delivery was accompanied by changes in obstetric practice. Writing in *The Lancet* in 1935, Eardley Holland said:

A striking change in the last 15 to 20 years is the remarkable widening of the indications for intervention during labour, and the great increase in the number of operative deliveries (induction of labour, forceps and caesarean section).[111]

He suggested that this was happening because the more frequent use of anaesthetics was slowing down labour and leading to an increase in the forceps rate and:

. . . the building of hundreds of little cottage and other hospitals giving to local practitioners who may possess neither the requisite judgment or the skill, the opportunity of performing caesarean sections and other obstetric operations.[111]

It may be that their greater ability to pay for the services of these practitioners accounted for the reverse social class gradient in maternal mortality among married women found in the *Registrar General's decennial supplement for 1931* which was published in 1938.[112] These data, shown in Table 2, had already appeared in 1937, in the last of a series of government reports on maternal mortality.[113] Contrary to the usual pattern, they showed higher mortality rates among women married to professional men than among those with husbands in semi-skilled and unskilled occupations.

Although these data were tabulated neither by place of delivery nor by birth attendant, evidence from a variety of sources suggests that, at this period, working class women were more likely to be delivered by midwives while a higher proportion of middle class women were likely to be delivered by GPs.[8] Many GPs were inclined to be impatient to use forceps or to do caesareans, for which most of them were inadequately trained.

Table 2

Mortality from puerperal causes per thousand live births, of married women, according to social class of husband, England and Wales, 1930-32

ICD code	Cause	Class				All married women
		I and II Pro-fessional	III Skilled	IV Semi-skilled	V Un-skilled	
140-150	All puerperal causes	4.44	4.11	4.16	3.89	4.13
140-141	Abortion*	0.50	0.56	0.56	0.57	0.55
142-150	Puerperal causes other than abortion	3.94	3.55	3.60	3.32	3.58
145	Puerperal sepsis+	1.45	1.33	1.21	1.16	1.29

Source: Registrar General's Decennial Supplement for 1931[112]

* excluding abortions certified as 'criminal'
+ excluding septic abortions

The 1937 report made a brief mention of a development which was to change the outlook for women contracting puerperal sepsis:

Since early in 1936 treatment of puerperal sepsis with Prontosil, a drug first introduced by Domagk in Germany in 1935, has been carried out in Queen Charlotte's Hospital Isolation Block. This treatment has been used solely for patients infected by haemolytic streptococcus and the results have been very encouraging.[113]

As Figure 10 shows, the maternal mortality rate as a whole and mortality attributable to puerperal sepsis fell sharply from the mid 1930s onwards. While this has been almost universally attributed to the use of Prontosil and other sulphonamides, the fact that the fall slightly preceded their introduction suggests that other factors may have also played a part.[114] For example, there were probably improvements in the standards of care given by midwives and the focusing of public attention on intervention by doctors without the necessary skills may have influenced decisions about whether to intervene and who should do so.[8] In addition, the pathology of the disease may have changed. Data based on notifications of puerperal fever show signs of a decline in mortality amongst women who were affected.[114]

Whatever the explanation, there is no doubt that sulphonamides were an effective treatment for puerperal fever in individual women. Thus when enquiries into maternal deaths were reorganised after the 1939-45 war, with responsibility passing from Medical Officers of Health to clinicians, different questions were asked and the idea that hospitals were potentially dangerous places was no longer current.

Confidential enquiries into maternal deaths

The first Confidential Enquiry into Maternal Deaths, covering deaths in England and Wales during the years 1952-54, looked at place of booking for delivery.[115] It classified women by where they were booked late in pregnancy or when labour began. Its judgments about 'unwise' booking for delivery at home or in a GP maternity home were based largely on clinical conditions observed in the antenatal period. It warned against:

The unwise acceptance for confinement at home or in small maternity homes of women with a known high risk in pregnancy, especially in the higher parities and older age groups.[115]

Subsequent reports based discussions of 'booking arrangements' on women's first place of booking, although the fact that some women booked to deliver at home or in maternity homes and others had transferred during labour was mentioned. Many women with 'no booking arrangements' were those who died as a result of illegal abortion, particularly before 1968 when the 1967 Abortion Act came into force.

The reports did not, however, attempt direct comparisons of risks associated with different places of booking or delivery. Instead, the second report emphasised 'the need for better selection of cases for hospital confinement based on the "priority" classes.'[116]

This approach was applied to analyses of both maternal and perinatal mortality and is described in the next section. It was used to establish criteria which were applied in subsequent reports[117] to judge whether booking for home or maternity home delivery had been made unwisely and thus set general criteria for booking for delivery.

The confidential enquiry report for the years 1979-81, was the first without a separate chapter on 'booking arrangements'. Of the 299 women who died, only four had originally booked to deliver at home, seven in an isolated GP unit and one in a private nursing home.[118] Place of delivery was not even mentioned in the report for 1982-84,[119] which was the last on deaths in England and Wales, or in the report on maternal deaths in the whole United Kingdom in the years 1985-87.[120] The latter did recommend that every consultant maternity unit should have a consultant obstetrician and consultant anaesthetist readily available to oversee the labour ward and that:

Any woman with a serious complication(s) of pregnancy must be transferred to a consultant maternity unit with appropriate facilities, including transport, to deal with this complication before her or her baby's life is threatened. Examples of such complications are worsening pre-eclampsia, preterm labour, and any serious medical or obstetric complication of pregnancy.[120]

The absence of explicit discussion of place of delivery in maternal mortality reports published in the 1980s is probably because the maternal mortality rates had been low for some years, as Figure 9 shows. As a result, the argument about place of delivery was now being conducted in terms of the mortality of babies.

The development of selection criteria

In the 1950s, successive Ministry of Health reports referred to rising demands for hospital delivery. This was first mentioned in the report for 1950-51:

> For the past 20 years there has been a progressive increase in the proportion of mothers seeking admission to hospitals for their confinements. The tendency was accelerated during the war, particularly in the rural areas . . .

> Housing conditions undoubtedly have a bearing but some areas with bad housing have lower hospitalisation figures than other residential areas where the conditions are good. Certain economic factors also play a part - whereas the woman confined in hospital has all her attendance and treatment free, the one confined at home may incur additional expenses for attendance, bedding, equipment and fuel, and has to provide her own food. While demands for hospital beds for acute cases, tuberculosis and other serious conditions cannot be met adequately in many areas, it is difficult to justify the provision of hospital accommodation for normal maternity cases simply because the mother prefers to have her baby in hospital.[50]

The problem was posed, therefore, as that of identifying the women most at risk for either obstetric or social reasons, and giving them priority for delivery in hospital where, it was assumed, they would do better.

A Ministry of Health memorandum published in 1951 recommended that:

Priority . . . should be accorded to (a) all cases in which there are medical or obstetric reasons in the widest sense of these terms (b) adverse social conditions, especially bad housing.[121]

It pointed out that:

(a) should not necessarily be regarded as including all primiparae, though admittedly a large proportion should be admitted . . .[121]

The Ministry of Health's reports on maternal mortality published in the 1930s had tabulated the deaths according to the women's ages and previous numbers of pregnancies. These were included in the discussions of social background. It was not possible to calculate mortality rates according to age and parity, however, because these data were not recorded at birth registration. In some areas such data were recorded by health visitors and these local data were used in the 1937 maternal mortality report.[113] In an analysis of these data, Percy Stocks of the General Register Office concluded that the maternal mortality rate was above average for women in their first pregnancy, declined for women in their second and third pregnancies, and was above average again for subsequent pregnancies.

The Population (Statistics) Act, which was passed in response to concern about the declining birth rate in the 1930s, enabled additional data relevant to fertility to be collected at birth registration. From July 1938, when the Act came into force, the parents' ages were recorded. If the parents were married to each other, the mother's previous number of live and still births by her current or any previous husband were recorded.

The immediate use of these data was to monitor trends in fertility. Later, after the war, they were used in a special study done by the Medical Research Council's Social Medicine Unit and the General Register Office. This looked at deaths under the age of one year among the 1.5 million children born in England and Wales in 1949 and 1950.[122] Information collected at death registration was linked to that collected at birth registration in order to investigate what were described as 'social and biological factors in infant mortality'. These included mothers' ages and parities, fathers' social classes and occupations, and parents' regions of residence.

Analyses of mortality by mothers' ages and parities[123], shown in Figure 11, were quoted in the Chief Medical Officer's report for 1955. Three so-called 'vulnerable groups' were identified:

1. Mothers over 35 bearing first babies have a high risk of stillbirth.
2. Mothers over 40 of any parity have a high risk of stillbirth.
3. Babies of young mothers with large families for their age have a high risk of death in the postneonatal period. This applies to the youngest mothers having a second or later child, and to mothers aged 20-24 having a third or later child, for example.[124]

A further analysis of the linked file data looked at the place of delivery of single legitimate live births in England and Wales in 1950 in relation to the 'social and biological factors'.[125] It also analysed the place of delivery of 'illegitimate' and multiple births in the County of London. It found that:

> . . . the proportion of births occurring in 'Institutions' conforms only in part with the risk of foetal or early infant death. In terms of parity the high mortality for the later births in large families (largely a function of maternal age, of course) is not matched by a correspondingly high admission rate to hospitals and nursing homes. This proportion decreases with maternal age, and women who have lost children have a lower admission rate than those who have not. Mortality rates increase as social class declines from I to V; admission rates decrease from social class I to IV and V.[125]

This was cited in the Chief Medical Officer's Reports for 1955[124] and 1956[126] as evidence of inappropriate selection of women for hospital delivery. The report urged hospitals to select, and GPs to refer to them, women in the 'vulnerable groups'. From 1957

Figure 11

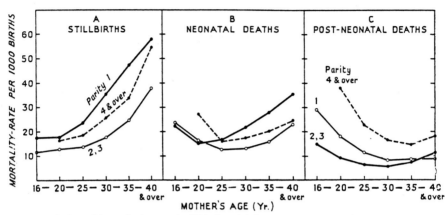

Fig. I—Variation with mother's age of stillbirth and infant-mortality rates (mothers of different parities compared).

Single, legitimate births in England and Wales, 1949. Stillbirth-rates, per 1000 live and still births ; other rates, per 1000 live births.

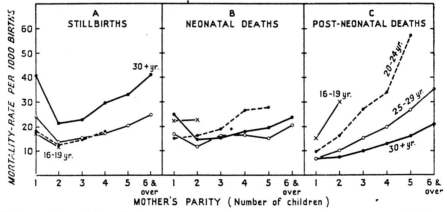

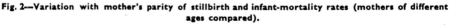

Fig. 2—Variation with mother's parity of stillbirth and infant-mortality rates (mothers of different ages compared).

Single, legitimate births in England and Wales, 1949. Stillbirth-rates, per 1000 live and still births ; other rates, per 1000 live births.

Reproduced from a paper by JA Heady, C Daly and JN Morris, the second of a series, entitled *Social and biological factors in infant mortality.*[123]

onwards, tables of numbers of births by mother's age, parity and place of delivery were published to monitor the extent to which this was happening.

Analyses of maternal death rates by age and parity were started in the Confidential Enquiry report for 1955-57[116] and extended in the following report, covering the years 1958-60.[117] As a result, the second of these reports made more detailed recommendations about selection for hospital care:

As an aid to the making of the best possible arrangements for any confinement it has been usual to list the indications for hospital care and responsibility on the following lines:-

1. All women who suffer from any illness that in any way impairs their general state of health. Obvious examples that come to mind are diseases such as valvular disease of the heart or diabetes.

2. Of equal or greater importance is grand multiparity. Parity greater than four is accompanied by a diminishing margin of safety and over nine the risk of death is very greatly increased.

3. All primigravidae over the age of 30, and multiparae over the age of 35 should be confined in hospital. The safety margin begins to contract over this age.

4. Any woman who has had abnormal previous pregnancies, labours or puerperia. In this respect the importance of previous toxaemia is generally recognized but the same cannot be said of previous post-partum haemorrhage.

5. For social reasons.

6. Primigravidae. Most women prefer to arrange for their first confinement to take place in hospital, not because they feel it to be dangerous at home, but because they feel it is safer in hospital - quite a different thing. After all, child-birth is a new experience and must be considered to be a trial.

7. Multiple pregnancy.

The first three of these should be regarded as absolute indications.[117]

These recommendations all tacitly assumed that women in the 'priority classes' or 'vulnerable groups' would necessarily do better in hospital. Neither the maternal mortality enquiries, nor the 1949/50 linked file study of 'social and biological factors in infant mortality' attempted analyses by place of birth. Indeed, the linked file study specifically ruled this out on the grounds that:

A direct comparison of the safety to mother and child in hospital delivery as opposed to domiciliary confinement, as at present organized, is vitiated because known difficult cases are normally booked for hospital and emergencies are rushed there. In fact, in any such comparisons, it is usual for the death rates to be higher in hospital than at home, though no informed person would adduce this particular fact as evidence that it is more dangerous to have a baby in hospital. On the contrary, in the present circumstances, there would be general agreement that, from a medical point of view, obstetrical cases which are likely to have material complications should deliver in hospital.[125]

It was therefore assumed that:

Groups of women whose babies are subject to a high 'perinatal' mortality rate - that is to say those who are more than usually likely to lose a baby by stillbirth or death in the first week - would benefit from hospital confinement.[125]

As a result there are no published analyses of differences in mortality by place of delivery within either low risk or 'vulnerable' groups, or analyses which relate to the considerable social class differences found in the study as a whole. Some later research did tackle these thorny questions and, in doing so, encountered the problems of bias referred to above.

The Maternity Services Committee, usually referred to as the

Cranbrook Committee, reported in 1959 that it had received a wide variety of views about the 'priority groups' for whom hospital care should be provided.[49] As far as primiparae were concerned, some groups had recommended that all should be admitted to hospital, while others advocated hospital delivery for all primiparous women aged over 30. The Committee's report commented, non-committally that:

> The arguments advanced for admitting all primigravidae were that in first pregnancies some abnormalities and complications of labour could not be foreseen during pregnancy and the admission of all primigravidae was therefore a precautionary measure which some felt to be necessary.[49]

On the other hand, the Committee's discussion of place of delivery gave equal emphasis to social need for hospital delivery.

Distinctions between different types of hospital were not usually made until the early 1960s, when they were used in analyses of the 1958 British Perinatal Mortality Survey.[127] Analyses of local data in the 1960s led to suggestions that all women who were in their first pregnancy or who had not previously has children should deliver in consultant obstetric units.[128-130] Whether they should do so became an issue.

The Department of Health and Social Security suggested in 1976 that general practitioner units should be phased out to make their resources available 'to other services which need them urgently'.[61] The House of Commons Social Services Committee's recommendation in 1980 that 'selection of patients is improved for smaller consultant units and isolated GP units'[63] further increased pressures to close them rather than to revise selection criteria. In the 1980s, the Department of Health adopted a policy that every woman should deliver in a district general hospital.[131] As a result, the safety of small maternity units in general has become the main issue.

Although mortality rates have decreased dramatically since the 1950s and 1960s, many of the same risk factors that were involved in selection then are still applied today. Moreover the issue has changed from selection for scarce acute hospital resources to selection for low risk maternity care in the context of choice. In the face of this, people working in primary care have suggested that the criteria need to be revised[132], and user groups have made similar demands.

Are age and parity still relevant?

Since the mid 1970s, it has become increasingly recognized that variations by mothers' ages and parities are difficult to interpret. This is because of social class differences which are associated both with the ages at which women begin childbearing and also with their overall standard of health. These are in turn associated with their chances of having a healthy baby. In addition, most published analyses of mortality by parity are restricted to births within marriage. This is now a major problem, particularly when interpreting data about births to younger women. In 1992, 31.2 per cent of all deliveries, 83.7 per cent of deliveries to women aged under 20, and 47.2 per cent of deliveries to women aged 20-24 occurred outside marriage.[35]

Tabulations of stillbirth and neonatal mortality rates for England and Wales by mother's age and parity are now published annually by the Office of Population Censuses and Surveys (OPCS). Stillbirth rates for 1990 showed the usual U-shaped pattern with the lowest rates for births to women of parity 1, who are women with one previous live or still birth within marriage.[68] The stillbirth rates for births to women having their first birth within marriage were lower than those for women having their fourth or subsequent birth. The same was true for neonatal mortality rates for babies born to women in their twenties. As with earlier analyses these are not based on successive pregnancies to the same women, and so may overestimate the effects of high parity.[133]

The patterns are very similar to those seen in analyses of the much higher death rates for 1949-50,[122,123] upon which the 1950s selection criteria were based. Thus the differentials persist despite the overwhelming extent to which women now deliver in consultant obstetric units.

Tabulations of mortality by age and parity are not published separately for each place of delivery. In any case, for isolated general practitioner units, the numbers of deaths are now so small that it would be difficult to detect any differentials that may exist. Marked differences between primiparous and multiparous women were found in a survey of all births at home in England and Wales in 1979, but rates for multiparous women were exceptionally low.[5]

The numbers of women dying in childbirth are now so low that the tabulation of maternal deaths by parity published in the Confidential Enquiry report for 1985-7 was based on deaths over 12 year period 1976-87.[120] Although this too shows the U-shaped pattern, with death rates being lowest among women in their second and third pregnancies, age differences were far wider, with rates for women aged 35 and over being more than twice those for younger women. Again, these patterns are similar to those seen in the much higher mortality rates which influenced selection policies in the 1950s.[115,116]

The most recent national statistics about complications experienced by mothers and their babies are those for 1985, the last year of the Maternity Hospital In-patient Enquiry (HIPE),[134] as its successor, the Maternity Hospital Episode System is still too incomplete to produce usable data.[135] Maternity HIPE was a 10 per cent sample of the 98 percent of all births in England which took place in NHS hospitals.

The HIPE data are based on all complications, including both those which needed attention from an obstetrician or paediatrician and those for which care from a midwife or general practitioner would have been appropriate. They show that first time mothers were more likely than women in subsequent pregnancies to have complications and that this was particularly true for older women. In contrast, there was very little difference in complication rates among their babies. Although the levels of these complication rates for women and babies are difficult to interpret, those for mothers show the same overall pattern seen in mortality rates.[136]

It should be emphasised that these data tell us that the proportion of women who may have problems varies from group to group. They can not tell us which individual women within any given category experience problems. A study in Wormeveer in the Netherlands has shown the success of midwives there in selectively referring to obstetric care during pregnancy both primiparous and multiparous women with problems which were diagnosed during pregnancy, but who initially booked with a midwife because they did not have known problems or an adverse past obstetric history.[137]

Mortality among babies and the place of birth

Since 1975, data collected at birth registration in England and Wales have been linked routinely to those relating to deaths of babies under the age of one year. Thus it has been possible to produce stillbirth and infant mortality rates for England and Wales subdivided by place of birth. These data are published annually by the OPCS in 'Mortality Statistics: childhood and maternity, Series DH3'.[68] Table 3 and Figure 12 present crude perinatal mortality rates for the years 1975 to 1991. Table 3 follows OPCS' convention of classifying NHS hospitals with a consultant obstetric unit as 'NHS hospital B' and those without a consultant obstetric unit, in other words 'isolated' GP maternity units, as 'NHS hospital A'. Some of the hospitals with consultant obstetric units also have GP maternity units and in recent years a few have developed midwife-led units. Figures for 'isolated' GP maternity units should be interpreted with caution, as some are incorrectly classified, and such errors have had a greater impact in the more recent years as the numbers of these units have declined.[138]

Before 1975 such information was available only from special one-off studies. Many of these were small scale local surveys, but two were the national birth surveys carried out in 1958 and 1970. Despite variations in scale and location these studies all revealed substantially lower perinatal mortality among births occurring at home or in isolated GP units, when compared with the rate among births in hospitals with consultant obstetric facilities.[48,139,140] In the last national study of this type, the 1970 British Births Survey, the perinatal mortality rate for singleton deliveries occurring in consultant obstetric units was 27.8 per thousand births compared with 4.3 for births taking place at home and 5.4 for births in isolated GP units.[140]

Table 3
Perinatal mortality according to the place of birth, England and Wales, 1975-91

		Place of birth				
Year	All	NHS hospital A	NHS hospital B	Other hospital	Home	Elsewhere

Total births

Year	All	NHS hospital A	NHS hospital B	Other hospital	Home	Elsewhere
1975	609740	43862	536091	9502	19504	781
1976	589979	45458	520856	8360	14667	629
1977	574664	39019	516894	7318	10940	493
1978	601526	35645	548796	6921	9608	556
1979	643153	32700	593964	7041	8904	544
1980	661007	27225	617485	7576	8162	559
1981	638699	22210	601740	7660	6560	510
1982	629870	21056	593868	7441	6969	536
1983	632765	19694	598799	7307	6443	522
1984	640461	18435	608178	7217	6149	482
1985	660062	16436	629714	7419	5955	538
1986	664567	14907	635741	7311	6064	544
1987	684934	16440	654614	7296	6018	566
1988	695959	14681	667314	7883	6468	613
1989	690961	9988	666127	7354	6963	529
1990	709398	11120	683032	7309	7363	574
1991	702471	9664	678309	6058	7832	610
1992	684056	9374	668609	4977	9235	621

Perinatal deaths

Year	All	NHS hospital A	NHS hospital B	Other hospital	Home	Elsewhere
1975	11716	218	10944	134	362	58
1976	10416	191	9785	118	272	50
1977	9717	202	9164	77	250	24
1978	9313	176	8821	67	200	49
1979	9402	122	8939	70	216	55
1980	8796	101	8381	68	204	42
1981	7521	63	7235	48	139	36
1982	7060	42	6782	56	140	40
1983	6561	41	6293	49	150	28

| | | Place of birth | | | | |
Year	All	NHS hospital A	NHS hospital B	Other hospital	Home	Elsewhere
1984	6440	37	6186	51	132	34
1985	6463	27	6231	57	129	19
1986	6338	35	6130	41	104	28
1987	6080	54	5853	44	101	28
1988	6061	24	7852	56	111	23
1989	5715	21	5530	49	92	23
1990	5716	16	5543	38	91	30
1991	5618	17	5418	43	114	26

Perinatal mortality rate

1975	19.2	5.0	20.4	14.1	18.6	73.8
1976	17.7	4.2	18.8	14.1	18.5	79.5
1977	16.9	5.2	17.7	10.5	22.9	48.7
1978	15.5	4.9	16.1	9.7	20.8	88.1
1979	14.6	3.7	15.0	9.9	24.3	101.1
1980	13.3	3.7	13.6	9.0	25.0	75.1
1981	11.8	2.8	12.0	6.3	21.2	69.6
1982	11.2	2.0	11.4	7.5	20.1	74.6
1983	10.4	2.1	10.5	6.7	23.3	53.6
1984	10.1	2.0	10.2	7.1	21.5	70.5
1985	9.8	1.6	9.9	7.7	21.7	35.3
1986	9.5	2.3	9.6	5.6	17.2	51.5
1987	8.9	3.3	8.9	6.0	16.8	49.5
1988	8.7	1.6	8.8	7.1	17.2	37.5
1989	8.3	2.1	8.3	6.7	13.2	43.5
1990	8.1	1.4	8.1	5.2	12.4	52.3
1991	8.0	1.8	8.0	7.1	14.6	42.6

Source: OPCS Birth statistics, Series FM1 and Mortality statistics, Series DH3.

Figure 12

Perinatal mortality by place of birth, England and Wales, 1975-91

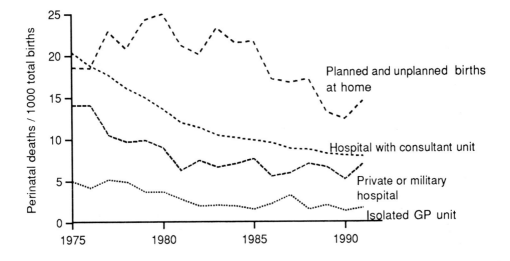

Source: OPCS Mortality Statistics, Series DH3[68]

Clearly, the findings of such surveys do not represent unbiased estimates of the risk of death attributable to the place of delivery, as no account has been taken of the complex biological, social and medical selection processes which influenced the choice of place of birth. Figure 13 shows diagrammatically the possible changes that can result from all these factors, and illustrates the complexities inherent in analysing any data about the place of birth.

Factors influencing selection can confound analyses by being related to both the place of delivery and the outcome. Thus, it is misguided to consider the effect of the place of birth on the outcome of pregnancy in isolation from the factors which lead different women to give birth in different locations, a point which was forcefully expressed by the British Medical Association in 1936:

Figure 13

Summarising possible movements between the actual and intended place of delivery

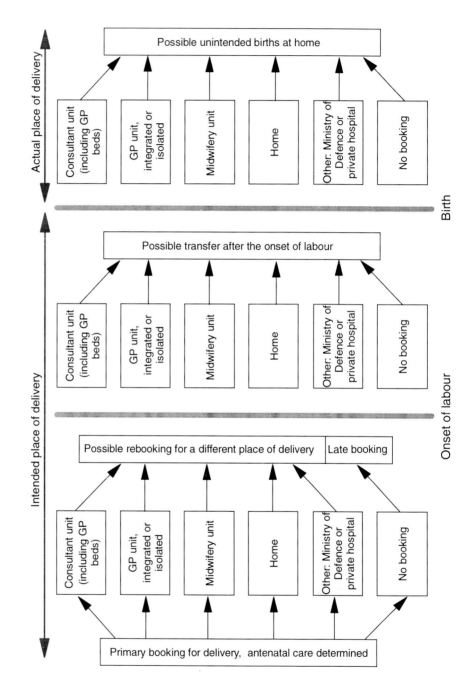

Maternity and its conduct are not concerned merely with attendance during the actual process of delivery, but comprise supervision from first to last - from the time that changes consequent upon conception manifest themselves until the return to normal some short time after childbirth. It is obvious that this whole period and event cannot be isolated from the rest of the health history of the mother, whether before, during, or after the period of actual pregnancy and parturition.[38]

When a decision about the place of delivery is taken, it is not merely the final phase of delivery that is decided, but also the particular system of antenatal care associated with it.[141]

Using standardised mortality rates

The technique used most often in attempts to control for selection biases has been to standardise measures of outcome for the different places of delivery to try to take account of variations in the proportion of women[142] or babies[143] possessing certain characteristics associated with an increased risk of perinatal problems.

Stephen Senn analysed data on all live births and stillbirths in Kent from 1973 to 1977. Of the 94,502 deliveries in the series, 79 per cent occurred in consultant units, 7.2 per cent in a GP unit and 8.3 per cent at home. The stillbirth rate for births in consultant units was approximately four times greater than that for GP units or home births. A birthweight standardisation involving 20 birthweight bands explained only part of this excess. The author concluded that 'an effect other than birthweight distribution, is required to explain differences in mortality according to place of delivery.'[143]

Unfortunately, deaths due to causes which could not have been influenced by the place of delivery were not removed from this analysis. These include congenital abnormalities incompatible with extrauterine life and intrauterine deaths which occurred before the onset of labour. Together these account for most stillbirths.[144] Consultant unit deliveries would almost certainly contain a disproportionate number of these deliveries. It is quite likely that they might have accounted for some or most of the observed differences in birthweight standardised stillbirth rates.

Marjorie Tew, a strong advocate of this approach, has carried out a number of standardisations using data from both the 1958 and 1970 British Births Surveys. Most of these involved standardising for single risk factors separately, a process she explained in detail in her book, *Changing childbirth*.[145] She has also analysed two weighted sums of a variety of risk factors. The Antenatal Prediction Score (APS) and Labour Prediction Score (LPS) were derived from analyses of 'data related to the biological and social factors constituting risk'[226] from the 1958 birth survey.[48] The scores were then reapplied to data from the 1970 survey.[146] The APS contained factors such as maternal age, parity, social class, previous obstetric performance and previous medical history and was intended to reflect the level of risk of perinatal problems during the antenatal period. The LPS contained the APS plus factors such as gestational length, complications during pregnancy and labour, fetal distress, presentation, twins and previous caesarean section and was intended 'to provide an index for predicting the outcome of labour'.[226] When perinatal mortality rates for hospital and domiciliary deliveries were standardised to adjust for the proportions of births in different risk categories defined by the Antenatal Prediction Score, the results recorded in Table 4 were obtained. This table is derived from an article in *The Lancet*[146] and subsequent correspondence.[147,148] Marjorie Tew concluded in her Lancet article that:

As measured by the APS, consultant units did indeed have a greater share of births at moderate and high risk than other places of delivery.[146]

In her subsequent letter to the editor she said:

This excess was sufficient to explain only a very small part of the excess mortality in hospital, as is shown by a comparison of the actual and standardised perinatal mortality rates. The difference between the standardised rates remains highly significant $(P < 0.001)$.[148]

Labour prediction scores for births grouped according to the place of delivery were not published in the original report of the 1970 survey but were later made available to Marjorie Tew. Her analysis of these data is reproduced in Table 5. These results show that at each level of risk, except for 'very high risk', perinatal

Table 4

Births and perinatal mortality rates by Antenatal Prediction Score, 1970

Place of delivery	Number of births	Perinatal mortality				
		Antenatal prediction score				
		0-2	3-7	>8	Actual	Standardised*
Consultant bed	11156	47.0	44.5	8.5	27.8	26.6
Integrated GP unit	526	65.0	32.9	2.1	9.5	10.5
Isolated GP unit	2584	64.9	32.7	2.4	5.4	6.0
Home	2706	69.1	26.8	4.1	4.3	4.8

* Using the indirect method.

Source: Derived by Marjorie Tew from analysis of data from 1970 British Births Survey[146,147,148]

mortality was significantly lower among births occurring either at home or in GP units than in hospital. In addition, the mortality of births at home or in GP units was uniformly low for those at very low, low or moderate predicted risk. This was not so for hospital deliveries where mortality appeared to rise as the predicted risk increased.

In Table 8.6 of her book *Changing childbirth*,[145] Marjorie Tew presented a revised version of Table 5. This time, she excluded births in GP beds in consultant hospitals. Doing so reduced mortality rates for births in GP units and at home and thus widened the differences between these and births in consultant units.

Commenting on the original version of Table 5 in her Lancet article, Marjorie Tew stated that:

> Unless some other factor can be found to explain these results from the obstetricians' own analysis of survey data, they must be interpreted as meaning that most infants do not benefit from active obstetric management and most of those already at higher risk benefit least.[146]

Table 5

Births and perinatal mortality rates (PNMRs) by Labour Prediction Score (LPS) and place of delivery, 1970

Level of risk	LPS	All births		Percentage of births at each score		PNMR per 1000 births	
		Number	Per cent	Hospital	GP Unit & home[+]	Hospital	GP Unit & home[+]
Very low	0-1	7488	45.9	58.7	41.3	8.0	3.9*
Low	2	3723	22.8	68.8	31.2	17.9	5.2**
Moderate	3	2273	13.9	76.6	23.4	32.2	3.8***
High	4-6	2417	14.8	84.0	16.0	53.2	15.5**
Very high	7-12	427	2.6	96.5	3.5	162.6	133.3

* $P < 0.05$ ** $P < 0.005$ ***$P < 0.001$
[+]   Includes general practitioner beds in consultant hospitals.
       Source: Analyses of unpublished data from British Births 1970[142]

Later on, in her book *Changing childbirth*, she commented:

> . . . the steeply rising mortality rate in hospital seems to confirm
> the frequently repeated dictum of the French obstetrician, Michel
> Odent, that the fetus already at increased risk is less able to
> withstand the stresses of obstetric intervention. It would seem
> that obstetric intervention, contrary to intention, does not in most
> cases reduce the stress of difficult labour for the fetus and hence
> the dangers for it of trauma and hypoxia.[145]

Is this interpretation of the findings valid? The nature of both the
data and the methods of analysis suggest that caution is required.

Firstly, the antenatal and labour prediction scores have not been
widely validated using other data sets.[149] In the 1970 survey, higher
antenatal and labour prediction scores were associated with raised
perinatal mortality rates. Their true predictive ability is not known,
however, and it may be this which accounts for some of the
unexplained differences between standardised rates.

Secondly, it has been suggested that analyses based on this type
of approach can be misleading because of subtle selection biases
for which it may not be possible to control, 'even when considerable
quantities of descriptive data are available for statistical
adjustment'.[144] There may be adverse factors and symptoms which
do not appear in risk prediction scores, but lead to individual
women being transferred to hospital care. Furthermore,
epidemiological studies, both in the perinatal[92] and cardiovascular
fields,[93] which have attempted to explain mortality differences in
terms of known risk factors have often failed to account for even
half of the observed differences in mortality.

Finally, it was not possible to exclude perinatal deaths resulting
from abnormalities incompatible with extrauterine life from these
analyses. As we have already indicated, these account for the
majority of stillbirths. Women thought to be at high risk of
delivering such a fetus or those who have been diagnosed
antenatally as carrying such an abnormality would have been
selectively referred to a consultant unit for delivery. Thus,
consultant units would have attributed to them a disproportionate

number of deaths resulting from causes unlikely to be influenced by the place of delivery.

Actual and intended place of birth

In addition to the difficulties posed by selection biases in choosing an appropriate place of delivery, analyses based on the actual place of delivery also fail to recognise that some women may not give birth in the place they had intended. For example, a women booked for delivery at home may, after an antepartum haemorrhage, be diagnosed as having placental abruption and be transferred for delivery in a consultant unit. Alternatively, a primigravid woman booked for delivery in hospital may fail to recognise her preterm labour and give birth at home unaided after a pregnancy of 28 weeks.

The extent to which this can happen can be seen in published tabulations of all births registered in England and Wales by actual place of delivery and birthweight. These are illustrated in Figure 14, which is based on data for the years 1986-88, because of missing birthweights in data for more recent years.[68] This shows that although very few low birthweight babies are born in isolated general practitioner units, there is a much higher proportion of very low birthweights among babies born at home, and an even higher proportion among babies born elsewhere outside hospital. This small group includes babies born in ambulances and in other places apart from the mother's usual place of residence, often unexpectedly.

Stillbirth and neonatal mortality rates, subdivided by birthweight, associated with different places of delivery show that for babies with birthweights under 2500g, stillbirth and neonatal mortality rates are higher at home than in hospitals with consultant units. These are likely to be births which occur at home unintentionally. Among larger babies, the differences are relatively small, but difficult to compare because of the small numbers of deaths of babies in this weight group born at home.[68]

Figure 14

Percentage of low weight births by place of delivery, England and Wales, 1986-88

Place of birth

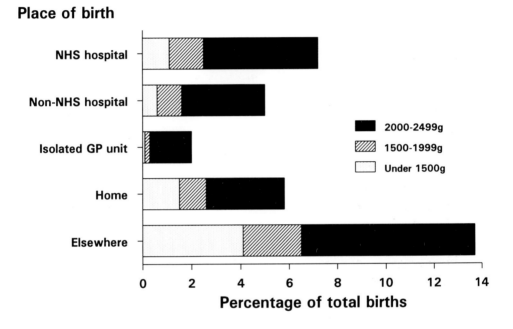

Percentage of total births

Legend:
- 2000-2499g
- 1500-1999g
- Under 1500g

Source: OPCS Mortality Statistics, Series DH3

A survey to determine the intended place of delivery at the onset of labour of all births occurring at home in 1979[150] found that, of these births, only two thirds had been booked for delivery at home. As Table 6 shows, the perinatal mortality rate for planned home deliveries was 4.1 per thousand births while for births at home which were planned to occur in consultant units it was significantly higher at 67.5. In all groups, mortality was lower in babies born to parous women, and it was particularly low for parous women having planned home deliveries.

Table 6

Births and perinatal deaths by intended place of delivery for all births occuring at home, England and Wales, 1979

Intended place of delivery	Births		Stillbirths and early neonatal deaths		Perinatal deaths per 1000 total births	
	No	(%)	No	(%)	Rate	95% confidence interval
Home	5917	(67)	24	(11)	4.1	(2.4 - 5.7)
Consultant Unit	1303	(15)	88	(41)	67.5	(53.9 - 81.2)
General practitioner bed	546	(6)	7	(3)	12.8	(3.4 - 22.2)
Unbooked	295	(3)	58	(27)	196.6	(151.3 - 242.2)
Not known	795	(9)	36	(17)	45.2	(30.8 - 59.7)
Total	8856	(100)	213	(100)	24.1	

Source: Home births survey[150]

Cumulative birthweight distributions, shown in Figure 15, show that the percentage of low birthweights was very low for women having planned home births, compared with the very much higher proportions among babies whose mothers intended to deliver in a consultant unit, or had no booking.

Figure 15

Cumulative birthweight distributions by intended place of delivery, for home births in England, 1979

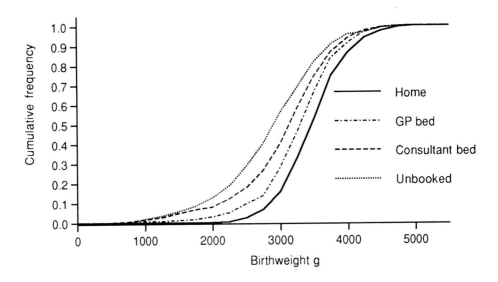

Source: Home births survey.[5]

Since 1977, as Table 3 and Figure 12 show, the overall perinatal mortality rate for births occurring at home has been higher than that for consultant units. It was suggested that this effect might be an artefact[151,152] and that with the decline in overall numbers of home births, an increasing proportion would be unplanned births at home.[150]

The results of the Home births survey,[150] together with the findings of other work[144] tend to support this hypothesis. The National Birthday Trust Fund survey of facilities available at the place of birth covered four separate days in 1984, when 1.0 per cent of births took place at home. This survey again found that two thirds of the births which took place at home were booked to occur there, while 28 per cent were booked to occur elsewhere and five per cent were unbooked.[153] Thus there had been little change since 1979. The decline in mortality, since the mid 1980s, in babies born at home suggests that there might have been a more recent decrease in the proportion which were not planned to occur at home.

As with analyses of maternal mortality, there is no general agreement about whether the intended place of delivery should be defined as that originally booked for delivery or that intended immediately before the onset of labour. Tabulations based on the place booked for delivery have two important advantages, however. Firstly, when women are grouped according to the place they originally booked for delivery it is possible to control for differences in antenatal care which may influence the outcome of pregnancy. Secondly, this approach also takes account of selection biases which arise when women are rebooked for delivery in different locations or are transferred to consultant units after the onset of labour.

Classifying births according to the place booked for delivery rather than the actual place of birth, as findings of four surveys summarised in Table 7 illustrate, tends to decrease the rate of perinatal death associated with hospital delivery and increase the rate for births booked for delivery at home or in GP maternity units. These findings are inconclusive in that, with the exception of the study by Louis Wood[154] for which raw numbers were not published, the differences between the mortality rates for hospital booked births and those booked for delivery at home are no greater than would be expected by chance. They also suggest that, at the time they were done, booking policies did not necessarily select high risk women for hospital delivery.

Selection in whatever form is not necessarily taken into account when births are grouped according to the place of booking. The study by Jean Fedrick and Neville Butler[155] illustrates how this problem can be overcome by making comparisons between relatively homogeneous groups of women. Their analysis of data from the 1958 British Perinatal Mortality Survey was confined to three relatively homogeneous groups of women with a low predicted risk of perinatal death. These were primiparae who remained normotensive, primiparae who were not normotensive and women of parity 1, 2, and 3 who were normotensive throughout pregnancy. This excluded:

. . . all women of parity 4 or more, those who had had a

previous stillbirth or neonatal death or liveborn baby of low birthweight (under 2500g), and those who had had previous toxaemia, antepartum haemorrhage, or delivery by caesarean section.[155]

Table 7

Perinatal mortality by place of delivery and place of booking in four studies in the 1950s and 1960s

Authors and location	Crude perinatal mortality rates					
	Place of delivery			Place of booking		
	Hospital	GPMU	Home	Hospital	GPMU	Home
Fedrick & Butler* Britain 1958[155]	11.46	10.7	6.80	8.70	12.00	9.25
Cookson, Gloucestershire 1953-1962[128]	46.92		7.59	28.57		24.12
Hobbs, Acheson Oxford 1962-1964[129]	26.0[+]		11.00[x]	19.00		20.00[x]
Wood L, Gwynedd 1946-1970[154]	52.00	8.40	18.90	36.70	23.70	19.70

*   See text for exclusions from the numerator and denominator of these rates

+   Includes a small proportion of deliveries for which there was no intended place of delivery.

x   GPMU and home combined

In this way, bias resulting from the selection of women at high risk for hospital delivery should have been reduced.

Although the authors reported that 'booking for NHS hospital delivery was associated with a consistently lower death rate ($p < 0.001$) than booking for domiciliary or some other type of confinement,'[156] this level of statistical significance was only achieved by combining death rates for all deliveries outside NHS hospitals within the three groups, and comparing these with the rates for NHS hospital deliveries. When the results for the three groups are pooled according to the booking for delivery, as in Table 7, there is no statistically significant difference between death rates for births booked for home or hospital delivery.[156]

Women transferred from home to hospital

Marjorie Tew has long maintained that it is only valid to compare perinatal mortality rates by actual place of delivery because women booked for delivery at home, but who give birth in hospital, are exposed to interventionist techniques employed in consultant obstetric units, which, she asserts, increase the risk of perinatal death.[157]

There is a considerable body of evidence, some of which is summarised in Table 8, showing that transfer to hospital, particularly in labour, is associated with a high death rate. Much of this information is based on small numbers of deaths and derived from surveys done many years ago. Some go back to the era when, as we have pointed out, women at high risk were not always referred to hospital. More recent information is not available either because it has not been collated or because it has not been published. Transfer to hospital usually arises because of the emergence of some problem such as, for example, placental abruption during late pregnancy or labour. This is likely to have an adverse effect on the outcome of pregnancy, and requires obstetric intervention. Thus, it is to be expected that babies born to women in this group would experience a higher mortality than those born to women delivering at home as planned.

Table 8

Perinatal mortality and home births: the studies in the 1950s and 1960s

	Perinatal mortality		
Author and period of study	Home births	Home births and labour transfers	All booked for home birth
Rees 1948-58[158]	21.5	24.1	26.3
Rutter 1961-62[159]	2.8	5.4	7.7
Hudson 1960-66[130]	5.4	6.8	8.9
Woodall 1950-69[160]	9.3	16.9	22.7

Marjorie Tew has, however, questioned whether this explanation for the higher mortality rates for those transferred is adequate. She argues that:

> When only a small proportion of bookings is transferred, it is likely to be made up of cases with very serious complications.[161,145]

If the proportion of women transferred increases, so the argument runs, a greater proportion of women with less serious complications and whose babies have lower risk of perinatal death will be included. Thus, as the proportion of transferred women increases so, she suggests, the gap between the mortality rate of those transferred and those remaining at home to give birth should narrow.

When assessing data from a number of studies,[162,163] Marjorie Tew finds that the proportion of women booked for delivery at home but transferred into hospital prior to the birth, to be high and yet the disparity between the perinatal mortality rates of those transferred and those remaining at home to be great. As these findings do not correspond to expectations, Marjorie Tew suggests that the high mortality rate for transfers is a consequence of obstetric intervention and concludes that transfer actually increases the risk of perinatal death.[157]

Even if it is accepted that Marjorie Tew's expectations are reasonable there are still flaws in this line of argument. For example, although cross sectional survey data indicate that the proportion of women transferred can vary considerably,[96,162,163,164]it is not at all clear whether there has been an increase in the proportion transferred. The results of an audit of women booked to deliver in an integrated GP unit but transferred to a consultant unit between 1970 and 1979 show a fairly constant transfer rate.[165] Another study of women delivering in Newcastle between 1960 and 1969 showed that the proportion of transfers increased over time, however. In line with Marjorie Tew's expectations, the perinatal mortality rate for transfers fell to a far greater extent than that for those remaining at home or those booked for and delivered in hospital.[96]

Marjorie Tew has used both direct standardisation and cause specific perinatal mortality rates to calculate expected numbers of perinatal deaths for transfers which could then be compared with observed rates. An example of direct standardisation can be seen in her analyses of published data from the Newcastle Maternity Survey.[96] Here, as shown in Table 9, perinatal mortality rates for home deliveries, hospital deliveries and women transferred for the period 1966-69 were applied to the proportion of births in each of these groups in the period 1960-62.

After standardisation, the adjusted or hypothetical perinatal mortality rates were lower than the actual or observed rates, suggesting that the overall mortality rate and that for births booked to occur at home would have been lower if fewer women had been booked for hospital delivery and fewer transferred from home to hospital. In order for this standardisation to be valid, however, the

Table 9

The composition of perinatal mortality rates, Newcastle-upon-Tyne, 1966-69

Deliveries	Actual			Hypothetical		
	Proportion of births 1966-69	Rate/ 1000 1966-69	Product	Proportion of births 1960-62	Rate/ 1000 1966-69	Product
Home	0.184	7.9*	1.5	0.447	7.9*	3.5
Transfers	0.048	56.4*	2.7	0.066	56.4	3.7
Hospital	0.768	25.9	19.9	0.487	25.9	12.6
All	1.000	24.1 = 24.1		1.000	24.1	19.8
Home bookings						
Home	0.791	7.9*	6.2	0.871	7.9*	6.9
Transfers	0.209	56.4*	11.8	0.129	56.4*	7.3
All	1.000	18.0* = 18.0		1.000	18.0	14.2

* Estimated using published data from the Newcastle Maternity Survey[96]
  Source: Reproduced from *Safety in intranatal care - the statistics*
      by Marjorie Tew[161]

composition of each of the subgroups and hence the relative risk of perinatal death in each would have to be assumed to have remained constant over time. Yet Marjorie Tew herself has suggested that this is not likely to have been the case.

In more recent work Marjorie Tew has suggested that the perinatal mortality for women transferred should not exceed that for those remaining at home by more than a factor of three. This was based on the overall perinatal mortality rates for all babies in the 1970 survey whose deaths were attributed to complications which would be likely to have led to transfer to hospital, had the woman been booked for home delivery. In fact, the perinatal mortality rate for babies born to women transferred was six times greater than for those remaining at home in the 1958 survey and 12 times greater in the 1970 survey.

Marjorie Tew has again inferred that the very elevated mortality rates in the transferred group are simply a consequence of increased obstetric intervention.[157] Her calculations not only exclude relevant but unknown data before labour but also are made without firm data about the reasons for transfer. More fundamentally, they are based on the assumption that the mortality associated with complications arising in women who intend to give birth at home, but were transferred, would be the same as that for women who intended to give birth in hospital. This ignores the possibility that any delay in obstetric intervention is likely to be greater in those being transferred from home and that this delay may well lead to a greater risk of death. Furthermore, the apparent increase in differences in the mortality for transfers in labour and babies born at home could simply have been because deaths which would have occurred at home in 1958 were occurring in hospital by 1970.

In response to Marjorie Tew, Jean Golding and Tim Peters, who had access to the individual records of data collected in the 1970 survey, were able to do a fuller analysis.[166] Although the place where women originally intended to deliver was not recorded in the survey, if a women did not deliver in the place she had originally booked, this was noted.

Raised perinatal mortality rates were found among babies whose mothers either delivered in hospital after having originally booked to deliver in any place elsewhere, or who had booked to deliver in hospital but actually delivered elsewhere. The same pattern was seen in mortality rates when women who had moderate or severe pre-eclampsia, a history of diabetes or any rhesus antibodies were excluded from the analysis. The authors admit that they were hampered by the exclusion from the survey of a question about women's intended place of delivery. They did not mention the importance of ascertaining whether the transfers took place antenatally or during labour.

A number of studies of transfers within the hospital system are relevant to the broader question of transfer from low technology to consultant care. A study in the John Radcliffe Hospital, Oxford, analysed transfers of low risk women who booked for shared antenatal care and delivery in the consultant unit with those who booked for community midwife and GP care with delivery in the integrated general practitioner unit. These analyses showed that the women transferred from the GP unit to the consultant unit as the result of some emergency arising during labour had outcomes which were as good as, or better than, those women who had the same initial low level of risk but were booked for delivery in the consultant unit.[91]

Leicestershire Perinatal Mortality Survey data for the years 1975-87 showed high mortality among babies whose mothers had booked for care in one of the isolated GP units but subsequently transferred to consultant care during the antenatal or intrapartum period. In 70 per cent of these deaths the baby either died before labour or had a lethal congenital malformation. Thus, for these babies the place of delivery would not have affected the outcome either way. In addition, perinatal mortality rates were adjusted for case mix and birthweight, using a different technique from Marjorie Tew, that of logistic regression. When this was done, the perinatal mortality rate attributed to immaturity among babies whose mothers were originally booked to deliver in isolated GP units but transferred to consultant care in the hospital with a neonatal intensive care unit was only 1.0 per thousand, compared with the unadjusted rate of 3.6. This highlights the importance of such adjustments for units providing neonatal intensive care. Most of this reduction is due to the adjustment for birthweight as hospitals with neonatal intensive care facilities admit a large excess of low birthweight babies.[167]

Analyses of data from the Scottish Perinatal Mortality Survey for the years 1986-1990 showed that there were 76 stillbirths and 55 neonatal deaths among babies born to women booked originally to deliver in isolated GP units.[168] Of these, 52 per cent, 41 stillbirths and 23 neonatal deaths, took place in teaching hospitals and 4 stillbirths were born in non-teaching hospitals. Stillbirths before labour accounted for 47 per cent and lethal malformations a further 16 per cent of these deaths of the transferred babies. As a result, antepartum stillbirth rates and mortality associated with lethal congenital malformations were lower among births occurring in isolated GP units than among hospital births. In contrast, neonatal death rates among babies born in the GP units with birthweights under 1500g were very much higher than among those born in teaching hospitals, with rates for non-teaching hospitals falling in between. These findings show the strength of using data about birthweights and cause of death rather than 'prediction' scores in retrospective analyses of place of delivery.

National data about transfers in labour in England should, in theory, be available through the Maternity Hospital Episode System. This system, which started in September 1988, should collect basic data about all women delivering in England. Items which should be recorded include intended as well as actual place of delivery and if these differ, whether the change resulted from a change of address or a decision taken for clinical or other reasons. A distinction should be made between decisions to transfer made during pregnancy, those made during labour and changes which 'occurred unintentionally during labour,'[169] a term designed to identify births after a very short and possibly unexpected labour, in which the woman did not have time to reach the place in which she had booked to deliver.

Unfortunately, the system has got off to a very slow start, and is still very incomplete. By the financial year 1989-90, the system contained records for only 55 per cent of births[135] and only about three quarters of all births in the financial year 1992-3 were covered.[170] Meanwhile, even the basic data, which used to be collected through Maternity HIPE, until it came to an end in 1985, are unavailable for subsequent years on a national basis. Although some data have been published, they are unreliable and are inadequate for analyses of actual and intended place of delivery.

On the other hand, the Maternity Hospital Episode System data which are collected can now be linked to information collected at birth registration. If it eventually proves possible to overcome the problems of incompleteness, and also to make a further link to

OPCS' infant mortality linked file, it should be possible to use the combined NHS and birth registration data to gain a fuller picture of the outcomes of pregnancy for women transferred during labour. The difficulties associated with interpreting these observational data will remain however.

Variations in hospital care

General practitioner obstetrics and the place of birth

The position of GP obstetrics within the place of birth debate is complex. Women giving birth under the care of a GP may do so at home, in an isolated or integrated GP maternity unit, or in a bed in a consultant obstetric unit. In addition, GPs may be called out to deal with obstetric emergencies outside hospital. This could happen, for example, when a woman who has concealed her pregnancy, is discovered by friends or relatives to be in the final stages of labour.[5] In reviewing published work on GP obstetrics it is pleasing to note that there has been a steady stream of GPs who have audited their obstetric work and published the results.[154,160,162,165,171-178]

One of the difficulties in classifying and interpreting these results, however, is the lack of standardisation both of outcome measures and of terms used to describe the various settings in which deliveries occurred. In particular, while the term 'integrated' has often been used to describe any GP unit which is on the same site as a consultant unit, more recently a distinction has been made between two types.[179] An 'integrated' unit has been defined as one which shares common wards and areas with a consultant unit while the term 'alongside unit' has been used to describe a unit which is functionally separate with its own ward and delivery area.

Another problem is that, because of small numbers, data have often been aggregated over several years during which the mortality rates are likely to have also changed. This makes interpretation even more difficult. Bias may also be a problem as the less conscientious GPs, who may have had poor results, are not likely to have taken the trouble to audit their practice in this way. Finally, it must be remembered that even though a woman might be booked to deliver under the care of her GP, the person most likely to be in attendance at the birth is a midwife.[83]

'Isolated' general practitioner maternity units

As was mentioned earlier, there has been a decline over the last decade in the number of deliveries in GP beds in hospitals. Much of this decline has resulted from the policy of closing isolated GP units. Between 1980 and 1990 the number of these in the United Kingdom halved from 212 to 106.[180] 'Isolated' GP units are characteristically small maternity units staffed entirely by midwives who are often community based, with GPs on call. These units are not on the same site as consultant obstetric units. A few are not far away but in many instances transfer to a consultant unit, if an obstetric emergency arises, may involve a journey of some distance. It is this lack of proximity to specialist obstetric and neonatal services which led a number of committees of enquiry, mentioned earlier, to question the safety of these units. Nevertheless, available data on the mortality among babies born in isolated GP units[154,160,162,167,168,181-184] calls into question the conclusion reached by the committees that these units are unsafe.

In statistics derived from birth registration published by the OPCS, these hospitals are classified as 'NHS A', that is, hospitals without a consultant obstetric unit. The percentage of births in NHS A hospitals and the attendant perinatal mortality rates for 1975 to 1985 are shown in Table 10. On the face of it these data suggest that delivery in an isolated GP unit is associated with a very low risk of perinatal death. It must be borne in mind, however, that only women thought to be at a low risk of experiencing perinatal problems would be booked for delivery in such a unit. Furthermore, perinatal deaths to women booked for delivery in isolated GP units but transferred to hospital during pregnancy or labour would not be included in these figures.

A further problem, also mentioned earlier, is that some of the units have been misclassified by OPCS due to deficiencies in the

Table 10

Perinatal mortality rates for babies born in isolated general practitioner units, England and Wales, 1975-91

Year	Number of births in IGPUs	Births in IGPUs as % of all births	Number of perinatal deaths in IGPUs	Perinatal mortality rate per 1000 births
1975	43862	7.2	218	5.0
1976	45458	7.7	191	4.2
1977	39019	6.8	202	5.2
1978	35645	5.9	176	4.9
1979	32700	5.1	122	3.7
1980	27225	4.1	101	3.7
1981	22210	3.5	63	2.8
1982	21056	3.3	42	2.0
1983	16694	3.1	41	2.1
1984	18435	2.9	37	2.0
1985	16346	2.5	27	1.6
1986	14907	2.2	35	2.3
1987	16440	2.4	54	3.3
1988	14681	2.1	24	1.6
1989	9988	1.4	21	2.1
1990	11120	1.6	16	1.4
1991	9664	1.4	17	1.8

Source: OPCS Mortality Statistics, Series DH3[68]

Note: In OPCS publications, isolated general practitioner units are labelled 'NHS A'

information supplied by regional health authorities.[138] Misclassification has posed greater problems in recent years even though the number of units has been relatively small.

The OPCS now publishes birthweight specific stillbirth and infant mortality rates by place of birth.   An analysis of stillbirth and neonatal mortality rates for 1986-88[185] showed that rates for babies born weighing less than 2500g in isolated GP units were lower than those for babies born in hospitals with consultant units and that the difference was greater than would be expected by chance.

This finding needs to be treated with caution because low birthweight babies form a lower proportion of all babies born in isolated GP units than they do of babies born in other places of birth. This probably represents further evidence of selection, with women expected to deliver a low birthweight baby being referred to consultant units.

The results of three surveys during the 1980s showed that overall perinatal mortality rates were low even when transfers in labour were taken into account.[186,182,176] In the first of these, an overall perinatal mortality rate of 5.2 per thousand births was estimated for women booked to deliver in isolated GP units in England and Wales in 1982.[186] This figure was based on survey data supplied by only 85 of the 131 units in England and Wales at that time, and so the possibility of bias cannot be ignored. In the other two studies, a perinatal mortality rate of 4.7 per thousand births was reported for all births intended to occur in an isolated GP unit in Penrith over the period 1980 to 1984[182] and a rate of 1.5 per thousand was reported for births intended to occur in a unit in Bristol between 1978 and 1985.[176]

In addition to being deemed unsafe, isolated GP units have generally been thought to be uneconomic. As a leader in *The Lancet* stated 'there has been a wide acceptance of the notion that, far from being beautiful, small is both ineffective and inefficient.'[187] In fact, as shown later when discussing costs, the relative cost-effectiveness of isolated GP units and other forms of hospital maternity units has yet to be established.

Irrespective of the academic arguments about safety and cost effectiveness, many of the local communities served by these isolated GP units seem convinced of their value and attempts to close them have often met with strong public resistance.[188] Both the Association for Improvements in the Maternity Services and the National Childbirth Trust have issued publications giving advice to groups formed to support the units and oppose closures.[189,190] More recently, the Association for Community-based Maternity Care was formed in 1989 by GPs and midwives who wanted to retain and promote this type of care.[191] A few years earlier, a survey in the Northern Region found that general practitioners were prepared to provide this form of care and made greater use of isolated GP units than they did of integrated GP units which were located on the same site as consultant obstetric units.[192]

Integrated general practitioner units

These integrated units, probably because of their close physical proximity to consultant obstetric units, have been less controversial than 'isolated' units. Judging by the published research, they have also been subject to less scrutiny, but in recent years, two evaluative studies have been published.

The first, an audit of women booked to deliver in such a unit in North Tees General Hospital in 1987, concluded that 'The general practitioner maternity unit provides a safe alternative for confinement in low risk pregnancies'.[193] Attention was drawn to the high rate of transfer to the consultant unit. Only 37 per cent of the nulliparous women and 65 per cent of the multiparous women booked for delivery actually gave birth in the GP unit. It was suggested that transfer rates could be reduced by having consultants attend women in the GP unit, if problems arose, rather than automatically transferring women to the consultant unit. The results of this study also indicated that apart from nulliparity, recognised risk factors were not good predictors of the need for transfer.[193]

The findings of the North Tees study are somewhat at odds with research undertaken in Bradford which focused only on women who booked for two integrated GP units in Bradford in 1988 but were subsequently transferred to consultant care. Twenty-nine per cent of those booked for GP care were transferred antenatally and 20 per cent after the onset of labour. The researchers concluded that 'Many of the problems that precipitated transfer were predictable and some were considered preventable' and suggested that high perinatal mortality among women booked for GP care necessitated 'tighter controls over the qualifications and experience of doctors participating in a fully integrated system of obstetric care'.[194]

In correspondence published in reply, the use of a crude perinatal mortality rate as an indicator of the quality of general practitioner obstetric care was heavily criticised because it does not take into account either socio-economic circumstances[195,196] or whether or not deaths are from causes which are considered to be preventable.[197] Subsequent correspondence warned of the danger of these findings being generalised elsewhere, when there were clearly particular problems of communication between professionals in Bradford.[195-199]

Curiously, both of these studies were undertaken by obstetricians, apparently without involving general practitioners. Apart from being open to the criticism of lack of diplomacy,[197-199] the authors of these studies also failed to make comparisons with data, to which they must have had access, about the outcomes for similar groups of low risk women booked to deliver under consultant care.

Comparative studies of GP and specialist obstetric care

A number of studies have attempted to compare perinatal mortality rates for women giving birth in different places under the care of a GP with those for women giving birth under the care of a consultant obstetrician. Earlier sections have looked at the differences in outcomes for home and hospital deliveries. The focus of this section is to consider specifically the institutional settings in which GPs take responsibility for women giving birth.

An analysis of 50,000 births which occurred in south west England between 1956 and 1967 found that perinatal mortality was higher for babies weighing over 1500g born in consultant units than it was for those born in GP units.[72] Similar results were found in an analysis of data for each health authority in England and Wales for the years 1978 and 1979. In these, when the proportion of deliveries in GP units was correlated with the perinatal mortality rate, no statistical association was found.[200]

Other research compared outcomes of deliveries in the late 1970s for similar groups of women in three different area health authorities. In two of these areas there were no GP deliveries, while in the third 34 per cent of deliveries took place in GP units. No statistically significant differences were found between the perinatal mortality rates for the three areas observed.[163] A study of perinatal mortality in Oxfordshire also 'failed to show that a high proportion of general practitioner deliveries constituted a major perinatal risk'.[201]

This apparently conflicts with the findings of a study in the Bath District.[202] Data in the Bath study were gathered prospectively for all women booked to deliver in a consultant unit, an integrated GP unit and seven isolated GP units during the period October 1984 to December 1987. Multiple births, births of babies with lethal congenital malformations and those weighing less than 2500g were excluded from the analysis.

The authors reported higher perinatal mortality rates in the isolated GP units than in the integrated unit and consultant unit and the chi-squared test showed that the differences were greater than would be expected by chance.[202] In this test, however, one of the cells of the table had an expected value of less than five which means that findings should be interpreted with great caution.[203] In addition, antepartum stillbirths were included in the analysis. This was despite the fact that, in the absence of further details about each case, the relevance of place of birth to these outcomes was open to question.[204] Furthermore, the authors failed to take account of risk factors other than parity.[205]

By the time the authors' paper was published, in September 1990, the district health authority had reviewed its policy and had decided to retain the isolated units, to provide additional equipment, and had appointed an additional consultant obstetrician to liaise with them. Data for the four year period 1988-1991 reveal no difference between the consultant unit and the isolated general practitioner units in the perinatal mortality rates for singleton babies born with birthweights of at least 2500g and without lethal malformations.[184]

For these reasons the authors' conclusion that it is a 'fact that it is not as safe to book for an isolated general practitioner unit as for a consultant unit' is not substantiated by their own research and is contradicted by more recent data. Indeed, of all the previous studies that have compared groups of low risk women in receipt of maternity care supervised by general practitioners with those receiving it from consultant obstetricians, only one has shown poorer outcomes for GP care.[206]

Selection of women for GP delivery

Who should give birth where, is a question which has always been at the centre of debate about place of birth. In an earlier section of this book we noted that the issue in the 1950s was how to ensure that 'priority classes' and 'vulnerable groups' had access to the limited numbers of hospital beds for which there was high demand. The untested assumption was that mortality for these groups would be decreased by institutional delivery.

As the number of consultant obstetric beds increased from the late 1950s onwards, the emphasis gradually began to shift from selection of high risk women for consultant care to identifying those at sufficiently low risk to be allowed a GP delivery. This process began by widening the criteria for selection of women for obstetric delivery. A number of papers published in the early 1960s questioned the selection criteria which had been drawn up at the time and considered whether all primiparous women, rather than only those over 30 should be booked to deliver in consultant units. The most influential of these analysed 5971 singleton births which occurred within marriage to primagravid women in the Oxford Record Linkage Study area from 1962 to 1964.[129]

This showed that there were no statistically significant differences in perinatal mortality between those booked to deliver in a consultant unit and those booked for delivery under GP supervision in a maternity unit or at home. One in six of the women booked for GP care were transferred to the consultant unit, either during pregnancy or after the onset of labour. The perinatal mortality for this group was more than three times the overall rate. There was some evidence that some higher risk women were being booked for hospital delivery, but the fact that this did not result in a higher perinatal mortality rate compared with deliveries under GP supervision suggests either that high risk women were receiving better care in hospital or that the selection was ineffective.

On the basis of their findings, the authors suggested that all primiparous women should be booked for delivery in consultant units. An alternative, and perhaps more appropriate conclusion might have been to suggest a review of the selection process.

Two other contemporaneous analyses showed that bookings for specialist hospitals may have contained a significant proportion of bookings for 'social reasons', such as inadequate housing, particularly amongst primiparous women[128] and that bookings for home births were made because hospital delivery 'was not generally available in the area'.[130] These factors may also have accounted for the possible inadequacies of selection found in the Oxford study. Another possible explanation is that GPs in areas which had GP units tended to book in to them women who should have been booked for consultant units.[58]

Table 11 summarises the findings of recent studies which have analysed transfer rates according to parity.[132,176,182,193] In spite of variations in initial selection referral policies, some consistent trends emerge. Firstly, transfer rates for primiparous women are consistently higher than those for multiparous women. Primiparous women are three to four times more likely to be transferred in labour than are multiparous women. It is also clear that compared with isolated units, transfer rates both antenatally and after the onset of labour are higher for women booked in integrated units. The authors of the study from Oxford commented that 'It would be relatively easy to reduce transfer rates by reviving the concept of consultation with the return of patient care to the referring general practitioner'.[132]

The numbers of deaths associated with transfers in labour reported in these studies are too small to interpret. Regrettably such data are not available nationally,[207] but there is a considerable body of data from earlier studies, showing that transfer from home or GP units to hospital, particularly during labour was associated with higher death rates among the babies. On the other hand, it is impossible to assess the extent to which the women concerned would have been selected for home or GP unit delivery today.

The complications which most commonly lead to transfer in labour in primiparous women are delay in the first and second stages of labour.[183,132] While transfer is always undesirable, it is notable that the majority of transfers are prompted by complications such as 'failure to progress', whose nature usually allows sufficient time for the transfer.

Table 11

Percentage of women transferred from isolated and integrated general practitioner units to consultant units, by parity.

Study and location	Parity	Antenatal transfer rate, per cent*	Transfer rate during labour, per cent[+]	Postnatal transfer rate, per cent[+]
Isolated general practitioner units				
Penrith 1980-84[182]	Primiparous }	20	15	} 1
	Multiparous }		5	
Keynsham 1978-85[176]	Primiparous	Not	19	Not
	Multiparous	available	5	available
Integrated general practitioner units				
Teeside 1962-88[193]	Primiparous	39	37	} 2
	Multiparous	24	10	}
Oxford 1981-84[132]	Primiparous	30	30	Not
	Multiparous	13	4	available

* Antenatal transfer rates are expressed as a percentage of all women booked for GP delivery units.
+ Transfer rates during labour and postnatal transfer rates are expressed as a percentage of all women intending, at the onset of labour, to deliver in the GP unit. They therefore exclude antenatal transfers.

The study in Bath District, discussed earlier in this chapter, did not detect any differences between perinatal mortality among babies born to primiparous and multiparous women booked to deliver in isolated GP maternity units. Rates for primiparous women booked for isolated units were higher than for those booked for delivery in the consultant unit and this difference was greater than would be expected by chance. This analysis failed to distinguish between antepartum and intrapartum stillbirths, however. This is important as the difference between the death rates attributed to intrapartum asphyxia was no greater than would be expected by chance.[203]

Selection criteria used today are still largely based on experience in the 1950s and 1960s. There is a need to evaluate whatever criteria are being applied[132] and at least two new studies plan to do this.[208,209]

Size of obstetric units

The allegation that the number of deliveries taking place in an obstetric unit is inversely related to the chances of a baby dying has been made for both general practitioner units and small consultant obstetric units. In 1980, the House of Commons Social Services Committee, as part of its report on *Perinatal and neonatal mortality*, published stillbirth rates for different types of obstetric units classified according to the number of deliveries in them each year.[63] These data, derived from DHSS' SH3 Hospital Return, are reproduced in Figure 16.

The Committee also noted the low overall stillbirth rate of 1.6 per thousand for births occurring in isolated general practitioner units and commented that 'This suggests that births in isolated GP units were already being selected fairly well for low risk status.'[63] Having said this, the Committee went on to express concern about 'the high stillbirth rates in the small consultant units, 4.57 in those delivering 200-499 births a year, and 7.74 in those delivering 500-999 a year'.[63]

It was this analysis of the data that led the Committee to recommend that:

Figure 16

DISTRIBUTION OF BIRTHS AND STILLBIRTH RATES BY TYPE OF UNIT.

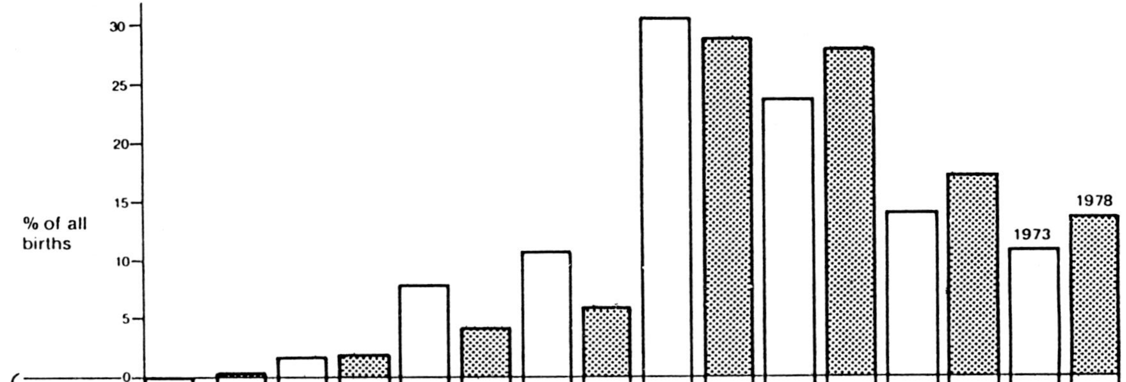

Reproduced from the House of Commons Social Services Committee report on *Perinatal and neonatal mortality*[63]

An increasing number of mothers should be delivered in large units; selection of patients should be improved for smaller consultant units and isolated GP units.[63]

The data published by the Social Services Committee took no account of differences between obstetric units of different sizes in the proportion of babies with low birthweights or congenital abnormalities. As the data only cover two years it is difficult to come to any firm conclusions about the relationship between the volume of deliveries carried out in an obstetric unit and the stillbirth rate. Nevertheless, even taken at their face value these data lend little support to the view that small units are less safe than those in which large numbers of deliveries take place.

For isolated general practitioner units, as the Committee itself pointed out, stillbirth rates were uniformly low. For units with both general practitioner and consultant obstetric beds the stillbirth rate for those with 200-999 deliveries per annum, although double that for isolated general practitioner units, was still low at 3 per thousand births.[63]

For consultant units there was a more consistent gradient in stillbirth rates in larger units. The stillbirth rate was highest in units with up to 2,000 deliveries a year. For units larger than this, the stillbirth rates remained constant regardless of unit size. Stillbirth rates for units with less than 1,000 deliveries a year were still significantly lower than those with a greater number of deliveries.

In a debate on maternity units in the House of Commons in January 1985[131] the then Undersecretary of State for Health, John Patten, quoted both the recommendations made by the Social Services Committee in 1980[63] and those made by that Committee in 1984, in a follow-up report in which it urged that:

> . . . the DHSS should do more to encourage regions, in the light of evidence available to them, to rationalise their maternity services in order to promote better standards of care as well as economy.[210]

He indicated that the Government's view still concurred with these recommendations. The criticism of small maternity units has been almost exclusively directed at those within the NHS, while some obstetricians continue to deliver women privately in small clinics, data from which are rarely published.

The National Birthday Trust Fund survey of facilities available at the place of birth[211] provided much useful descriptive information about maternity services in the United Kingdom in the early 1980s. Unfortunately sufficient funds were not available to link this information with details about stillbirths and infant deaths derived from registration particulars. This meant that the opportunity to analyse the association between lack of appropriate obstetric, paediatric and anaesthetic services and mortality was lost.

Studies of perinatal outcome according to size of unit in other developed countries tend to suggest that babies weighing less than 2500g at birth have a better chance of surviving in large obstetric units.[212-214] Analyses of data from Scotland shows that these babies have enhanced chances of survival if they are born in teaching hospitals.[168] There is even some suggestion from abroad that mortality for babies weighing 2500g and over is lower if the birth takes place in a smaller unit but this was not found to be the case in Scotland.[168]

'Domino' Schemes

The term 'domino' is derived from the phrase '*dom*iciliary *in* and *o*ut'. The first time it appears to have been used was to describe a community obstetric project set up in West Middlesex in 1971.[215] In this scheme, intended to 'integrate' community midwifery with hospital practice, community midwives were able to book low risk women for a hospital delivery. As well as doing the antenatal care themselves, midwives accompany the women into hospital after the onset of labour and take responsibility for the delivery. If there are no complications, women can then go home just a few hours after the delivery.

When this scheme was first described in 1975 it was claimed to be 'an entirely new style of practice'. In fact, the idea had been floated some 15 years before the West Middlesex scheme began[56] and reports of two schemes which predated it had been published. The first report was in the *Chief Medical Officer's report for 1963*.[216] This described a system in Luton where women were discharged as soon as they were 'fit to be moved' after delivery. This had apparently been started because of a shortage of maternity beds. It was given as an example of one of three types of early discharge schemes. The other two kinds were discharge after 48 hours or after seven days.

The only published statistics about mortality in a short stay scheme appeared in 1970. These came from an experimental system in Salford which had been started in 1967.[217] After its first two years in operation, 641 women had been admitted. Of these, four women had to be readmitted after discharge following postpartum haemorrhage, 47 were transferred to a specialist unit during labour and 14 after delivery. Thirteen babies were transferred to a special care baby unit. Altogether there were four perinatal deaths, one of which was a stillbirth after a forceps delivery, and one a macerated second twin. Two neonatal deaths were attributed to congenital heart disease. Thus, the overall perinatal mortality rate was 6.24 per thousand births.

Given that 'domino' schemes are often promoted as the ideal compromise between home and hospital delivery it is surprising that there has been so little evaluation of them, particularly as early discharge is increasingly becoming a routine policy. The only recent study was a randomised trial which compared the outcomes for women delivering in St George's Hospital Tooting, as part of a domino scheme entitled 'Know your midwife', with those for women receiving the standard consultant obstetric care given at the hospital.[218] The results of this trial are described in the next section.

Midwifery and the place of birth

As midwives we think we work hard, we think that we give a
valuable service with good outcomes, we think that we provide an
economical service; but thinking is very far from knowing, when
we are asked to produce statistical evidence of our achievements,
we struggle to do so, because audit which is discretely related to
midwives work is not routinely undertaken. [219]

Julia Allison, Sir William Power Memorial Lecture, 1991

The majority of babies born in the United Kingdom have always
been delivered by midwives, a fact often overlooked both by policy
makers and research workers alike.

Since the first edition of *Where to be born?* was written there have
been important developments in midwifery with greater recognition
of the actual and potential role of midwives. One consequence of
this has been a substantial increase in the amount of published
research conducted by midwives,[220] although only a small proportion
of this has been concerned with place of birth. In addition,
changing views of maternity care during the latter half of the 1980s
led to the emergence of a number of new settings for birth, often
described as midwife-led units.

The defining characteristics of these units, as their name suggests,
is that they are run entirely by midwives. Obstetricians and general
practitioners may refer women to such a unit for delivery but
midwives take full responsibility for women delivering there, with
medical assistance being sought when a midwife deems it
appropriate. In some respects, these principles are not new but
echo those set out for 'maternity homes' in the 1920s.[24]

As midwife-led units are a new phenomenon there are no national data on how many exist or the numbers of deliveries which take place in them. Rather like general practitioner units, some appear to be 'integrated', that is on the same hospital site as consultant obstetric units[89,218,221] while at least one that we are aware of is on a hospital site which does not have a consultant obstetric unit.[222]

At the time of writing, many evaluations are being planned, while one in Bournemouth is still under way,[222] the results of a second evaluation in Aberdeen[221] are likely to published shortly and the results of an evaluation in Leicester are already published.[89] In the Aberdeen evaluation, low risk women were invited to take part in the study and then randomised at their booking visit to book for delivery in a midwife managed unit or in the consultant supervised labour ward.[221]

The evaluation of the third, the 'Home from home' scheme in the Leicester Royal Infirmary, was also a randomised trial.[89] It compared 2,304 women assigned to this midwife-led scheme with 1,206 similar women allocated to consultant-led care. This showed few significant differences in adverse events before, during or after delivery and no difference in the percentages of mothers and babies discharged home alive. In general, women allocated to midwife-led care were more satisfied with care given antenatally and during labour and delivery.

In a trial, consent is usually obtained prior to randomisation into experimental and control groups. This was done in the Aberdeen study, but in Leicester all women deemed at the antenatal booking clinic to be suitable candidates for midwife-led care were randomly allocated to receive either the normal consultant-led care or the experimental midwife-led scheme of care. Consent was only sought from those in the experimental group, however. Women who had been allocated to the consultant-led scheme were not given the opportunity to say whether or not they wished to participate in the trial. This led to 'contamination' in the experimental group because 189 or eight per cent of the women in it said that they did not want midwife-led care. As they had already been allocated to this group before being asked to take part, outcomes for these women were attributed to midwife-led care. On the other hand, as women allocated to consultant-led care were not asked for their consent there was no comparable group of women who refused consultant-led care and opted instead for midwife-led care.

The trial appears to have been designed with an expectation that approximately 50 per cent of women booked for midwife-led care would be transferred. Thus, for every one woman randomised to consultant-led care two were allocated to midwife-led care. This anticipated level of transfer actually occurred. Twenty three per cent of the women allocated to midwife-led care were transferred antenatally, 20 per cent were transferred during labour and a further two per cent were transferred after delivery.[223] Hypertension, gestation of over 41 weeks and vaginal bleeding were the most common reasons for antenatal transfer and meconium stained liquor and failure to progress were the most frequent reasons for transfer during labour.

Interestingly, for three per cent of antenatal transfers no reason was recorded. Furthermore 28 per cent of antenatal transfers and 15 per cent of intra and post natal transfers were grouped together as having 'other' reasons for transfer. The authors of the report of the trial commented that:

> In a number of cases, no obvious or an insignificant reason for transfer was noted. This was usually because the women had been admitted to specialist care before 37 weeks, or because she had been referred back to a clinic by a general practitioner or midwife. Women tended to be retained for specialist delivery by default.

This suggests that the transfer rate need not have been as high. Nevertheless, the authors conclude that 'even though only half of hospital bookings are suitable for such midwifery-led care and bearing in mind that half of these will return to specialist care, it can be seen that approximately 25 per cent of mothers initially referred can achieve delivery without the assistance of doctors.'

The word 'midwife' means 'with woman' and the professional role of the midwife in assisting and supporting women in childbirth has meant increasing emphasis being placed on the continuity of care.[224] The move from home to hospital together with changes to the pattern of ante-natal and post-natal care has in many cases led to increasing fragmentation.

The 'Know your midwife' scheme was set up in St George's Hospital, London to try to increase continuity of care for women delivering in a consultant unit in a large London teaching hospital. In order to reduce the number of staff women saw during their pregnancies, a team of four midwives was established to provide complete antenatal, intrapartum and post-natal care. To evaluate the effectiveness and practicability of the scheme it was introduced on a trial basis. Between April 1983 and March 1985, low risk women booking at the hospital who wished to enter the trial were randomly allocated to the scheme or to the normal pattern of consultant care. Data relating to women who had transferred to consultant care during pregnancy or labour were analysed in the 'Know your midwife' group.

The scheme did produce greater continuity of care. Fewer care givers were seen during pregnancy, and in nearly every case the midwife who was with the woman throughout her labour and delivery was one of the team of four. Women in the 'Know your midwife' scheme were more likely report to feeling in control during labour, and they received less analgesia. Labour was longer for women in the 'Know your midwife' group. This may have been because fewer labours were augmented but could also reflect different definitions of the onset of labour. A smaller proportion of women in this group had episiotomies but this was offset by a higher rate of vaginal tears. Six weeks after the birth women in the 'Know your midwife' group had much more positive recollections of labour. They felt better prepared for child care and more able to discuss any difficulties they were experiencing.[218]

There were more perinatal deaths to women in the 'Know your midwife' group but these were not related to factors in the scheme. The difference in mortality rates was no greater than would have been expected by chance, although this may have been a function of the small numbers of women in each group.

The type of care provided by midwives in 'domino' schemes was available to much larger numbers of women during the heyday of domiciliary midwifery, between the inception of the National Health Service and its reorganisation in 1972. The difference then was that for these women, all care, including intrapartum care, took place outside hospital, much of it in women's own homes. Julia Allison, a midwife from Nottingham, has done a historical audit of the caseloads of district midwives in the city during this period.[219]

Some of her data are shown in Table 12. These show that stillbirth and neonatal death rates in Nottingham fell at the same pace for home and hospital births. This is consistent with findings for a similar time period in Newcastle upon Tyne.[96]

Table 12

Births, stillbirths and neonatal deaths in Nottingham by place of birth, 1955-72

| | Total births Number | | Stillbirths and neonatal deaths Number | | Rate/1000 births | |
Year	Home	Hospital	Home	Hospital	Home	Hospital
1955-57	8011	7770	160	445	20.0	57.3
1958-60	8672	8372	138	484	15.9	57.8
1961-63	9354	9172	128	524	13.7	57.1
1964-66	8062	10406	90	554	11.2	53.2
1967-69	5987	11409	71	431	11.8	37.8
1970-72	3682	11162	42	343	11.4	30.8
Total	43768	58291	629	2781	10.0	50.0

Source: Allison J, *Midwives step out of the shadows* [219]

Data from Nottingham also show mortality rates for births at home to have been substantially lower than those for births in hospital. The death rates in hospital might have been expected to be higher because of the selective referral of women at high risk of complication but, as noted earlier, not all high risk women were able to obtain a hospital birth at this time.

It is perhaps more surprising that death rates for home births were so low, particularly as Julia Allison estimates that over half of the women in Nottingham giving birth at home fell outside today's criteria for home birth on grounds of age, parity and maturity of pregnancy. In addition, mortality among babies born to women who had no antenatal care and were unbooked for delivery and those who were booked for delivery in hospital but had an un-planned birth at home because of a precipitate labour were in-cluded in the rates for home births. Such births were classified as a BBA meaning 'born before arrival' either at hospital or in the ab-sence of a qualified birth attendant. Many of these births would have had a considerably increased rate of perinatal death.

The vast majority of midwives in the United Kingdom practice within the NHS but a few work either in private hospitals or as independent practitioners. Many of those practising independently are midwives who had become disenchanted with the way in which maternity services were provided within the NHS, finding them to be over medicalised, fragmented, unfriendly to women and failing to utilise the full range of skills possessed by midwives.[225]

Deliveries undertaken by independent midwives are not separately identified in national data but an audit of their work for the period 1980 to 1991 has recently been published.[225] Unfortunately, only 58 per cent of the 73 midwives known to have been practising during that period supplied information for the audit and therefore the findings may not be truly representative. In particular, response was low among midwives who had gone to independent practice relatively recently.

The audit population was defined as all women whose birth was attended by an independent midwife. Thus, women who may have received antenatal care from an independent midwife but who for some reasons were delivered by some other professional were not included.

One thousand two hundred and eighty-five births were included in the audit. During the period reviewed, the perinatal mortality rate for the audit population was 7.7 per thousand while the national rate for England and Wales fell from 13.3 in 1980 to 8.0

in 1991. Three quarters of the women gave birth at home. The other quarter were transferred into hospital at some time during labour. Just over two thirds of transfers to hospital were unplanned. This constituted 17 per cent of all the births audited. Almost half of the mothers in the audit population were nulliparous and 63 per cent were aged 30 or over.

As this edition goes to press, further developments in midwife-led care are getting under way or are at the planning stage in different parts of the country. It is encouraging to hear of plans which are being made to evaluate some of these changes as they occur.

Morbidity in women and their babies and the place of birth

With the reduction in stillbirths and neonatal mortality rates, epidemiological interest has become increasingly focused on morbidity and how this might be a possible indicator of the quality of obstetric care. As was mentioned earlier there is a wide range of morbidity which could be considered. For women there are rare but life threatening conditions, notably post-partum haemorrhage, for which prompt access to medical facilities is required. On the other hand there is extensive morbidity among women associated with conditions which are not life threatening but can cause considerable pain, sometimes over long periods.[69] For babies both illness after birth and health later in childhood may be associated with the care given at birth. Studies of morbidity in relation to the place of birth are few and often do not cover all these aspects of morbidity. Nevertheless they merit consideration within the context of this review. Because there are so few of them, some studies from abroad have been included for comparative purposes.

The 1970 British Births Survey compared babies born in different settings and defined as unfit. Babies born at home suffered more often from jaundice and minor infections than those born in NHS hospitals and GP maternity units. Conversely, a larger percentage of babies born in these institutions had the more serious conditions such as congenital malformations, fits, cerebral signs and respiratory difficulties[226] Similarly, a study of cerebral palsy among children born in the Northern Region of England between 1960 and 1975 showed lower rates of cerebral palsy among children born at home or in small units without resident staff than in children born in consultant units, even when differences in the birthweight distribution were taken into account.[227]

A study of 1,692 women at low risk who had babies in Groningen Municipality in the Netherlands in 1981 showed that women who opted to give birth at home experienced fewer complications during pregnancy, labour and the puerperium than those who chose to give birth in hospital, even when parity was taken into account. Women in the study population initially had a free choice as to where they gave birth. This could either be 'in hospital' with a one day or a seven day stay, or at home. If any abnormality arose during pregnancy in those booked for delivery at home, their booking was changed to hospital. In babies born without complications, morbidity leading to referral to a special care nursery was lower in those born at home than in those born in hospital.[228]

The findings of the British Births Survey, that babies born at home suffered more minor infections than those born in hospital, are unusual in that the risk of infection is generally accepted as being higher for babies born in hospital. An earlier study compared the outcomes of 233 home deliveries and 270 deliveries in hospital. When babies described as 'premature' and those with jaundice and congenital abnormalities were excluded, babies born at home were found to be less liable to contract infections during their first 28 days of life.[229] This study also found that 46 per cent of women giving birth in hospital had either a perineal tear or an episiotomy compared with 31 per cent of those who gave birth at home.

An analysis of all births occurring at home in Cardiff between 1970 and 1979 found mortality and morbidity among the 315 planned home births to be very low.[144] This included eight babies born to women booked for delivery at home but transferred into hospital prior to delivery. Only two babies died, both before the onset of labour. One death was associated with rhesus isoimmunisation. The cause of the other stillbirth was unknown. The only notable morbidity was respiratory distress. This developed in two babies born with low birthweight, one delivered by caesarean section. In this instance, the mother had been transferred to hospital after an intrapartum haemorrhage.

In contrast, there were 13 perinatal deaths among the 159 unplanned home births. This group also suffered a considerably higher rate of respiratory distress. The rate was 44.0 per thousand unplanned home births compared with that 15.9 per thousand planned home births. There were also 25 reports of hypothermia, 8 of cerebral irritation and pneumonia among the 159 unplanned home births.

In addition to details of the intended place of delivery for all mothers giving birth at home in England and Wales in 1979, midwives completing questionnaires in the Home Births Survey were asked to report whether there was any abnormality present in the baby at birth. Overall, far fewer abnormalities were reported for babies whose births were planned to occur at home.[5]

As a further way of obtaining data on morbidity, midwives also reported whether or not mothers and babies had been transferred into hospital after delivery. Many of the women whose births were not intended to occur at home were transferred into hospital afterwards as a matter of routine. Of those deliveries planned to occur at home, 3.5 per cent of babies were subsequently transferred to hospital. The reason for more than half of these transfers was for the babies to be with their mothers in hospital. Of the women who gave birth at home as planned, 2.8 per cent were transferred into hospital after delivery, and 46 per cent of these had retained placentae.[5]

Another approach to studying the morbidity of women giving birth at home has been to review the complications of low risk women who gave birth in hospital. In an exercise of this type, the maternity records of 1,015 deliveries which occurred in a Liverpool hospital in 1978 were reviewed. Of these, 278 or 27.4 per cent were considered to have been suitable for home delivery at the time of booking. Fifteen per cent of those thought suitable to have been booked for a home delivery experienced complications during the antenatal period which would probably have resulted in a change of booking. A further 12 per cent had complications during labour or the first five days after delivery and 16 of the babies required specialist paediatric care at or immediately after birth.[230]

The results of this study do not, of course, represent accurate estimates of the morbidity and mortality associated with booking for a home delivery, as all the women included were actually booked and delivered in the maternity unit of a district general hospital. Thus the findings reflect the risks associated with the type of care actually received. Furthermore, as this study reviewed the women retrospectively rather than following them prospectively, the possibility of bias in determining who would have been suitable for a home delivery cannot be excluded.

The findings of these descriptive studies are of interest, but no attempt has been made to control for selection biases. This means that it is not possible to assess the extent to which differences in morbidity can be attributed to differences in the place of birth.

Three other studies have attempted to contrast morbidity in similar populations of women at low risk who gave birth in different settings. A study in Oxford in 1978 compared the outcomes for low risk women booked for delivery either within a system of consultant based shared care or with community midwife and GP-based care.[91] It was found that in babies born to nulliparous women, the proportion who had low Apgar scores and were intubated was lower in those booked for delivery in the GP unit. The use of epidurals and pethidine was considerably higher in nulliparous women booked for delivery in the consultant unit under the shared care system.

Although the authors concluded that it was not possible to say which procedures used in the consultant unit might have accounted for observed differences in the babies, they did suggest that the use of analgesia and perhaps anaesthesia merits further attention.[141] A follow-up study done in 1981 found fewer differences between patterns of care in labour in the two systems, but it covered only 171 women and the differences between the groups were no greater than would be expected by chance.[231]

Similar results have also been reported by a general practitioner who undertook a prospective survey of 202 women booked for delivery at home and a similar group of 185 women booked for delivery under consultant care during the period 1978 to 1983. The induction rate in women booked for hospital delivery was more than double that for women booked to give birth at home. In addition, there was a higher rate of episiotomies and second degree tears and more Apgar scores of 7 or below among women who were booked for hospital.[232]

A retrospective comparison has also been made between 185 low risk women intending to give birth in an isolated general practitioner maternity unit and a comparable group of women who gave birth in a consultant unit.[176,175] Greater use of pethidine was made in the general practitioner maternity unit. This may have outweighed the use of epidural anaesthesia in the consultant unit.

Labour was significantly longer for women in the general practitioner group, where significantly few labours were augmented, but the authors suggest that this may have been due to a difference in the way the onset of labour was defined in the two units. There were no statistically significant difference in rates of episiotomy and tearing between the two groups. Post partum haemorrhage and anaemia were more common among women in the general practitioner group, although this may have been due to recording bias. Meconium staining and intubation were more common in babies born in the consultant unit but there was no difference between groups in the proportions of babies in each group with Apgar scores below six at one minute after birth.

A study in the United States matched 1,046 women who, immediately before the onset of labour, intended to give birth at home, with a similar group of women intending to give birth in hospital.[233] The women were matched for age, education, socio-economic status and obstetric risk factors. Although the episiotomy rate was nine times higher among women who delivered in hospital, the proportion who had serious lacerations was higher than among women who gave birth at home. A significantly greater proportion of babies born in hospital had birth injuries, neonatal infections, respiratory distress lasting 12 hours or more and non-congenital neonatal complications. There were, however, no statistically significant differences in mortality or neurological impairment.

Thus, studies from the United Kingdom, in particular those using a comparative approach, are few in number, but tend to suggest that the more common but non life-threatening types of maternal and neonatal morbidity are more common in hospital settings. There are too few data to compare the settings in respect of more serious but uncommon types of morbidity. There is clearly a need for up to date comparisons based on larger numbers of women and babies.

Costs of maternity care

Costing maternity care is a long standing concern. For example, in his book *Deaths in childbed* published in 1879, Aeneas Munro set out a scheme for a model maternity institution consisting of 'a lying-in hospital and a training school for medical men and nurses or midwives.'[19] Introducing his estimates of costs and how to meet them, he commented that 'there is no subject more pressing for attentive consideration then that of how these institutions are to be maintained. The cost is unequally borne. Humane and thoughtful men, and women too, have always borne the burden and the heat of the day in this battle. But the saying "we must draw the line somewhere" must force itself upon them even when the purse is deep and large.'[19]

Over the past twenty years, costs have become an increasingly dominant issue in discussions about provision of maternity care. Unfortunately, there has not been a corresponding increase in collection of information on the costs of birth in different settings.

Claims are often made that small maternity units are uneconomic and since the early 1980s many have been closed on the grounds of cost. It has also been asserted that home births are expensive in comparison with births in hospital, although in 1992 the Department of Health admitted, in response to a parliamentary question, that it did not have comparative information about the costs of normal births in hospital and at home.[234]

When Miranda Mugford reviewed evidence about the costs of delivery in different settings, she found that little was available. Most relevant studies had been done many years ago.[235] Some were published in health authority papers presented to justify closures of GP units and these seemed to have given little thought to the question of what methodology was appropriate for economic appraisal of alternative policies.

The study of a week's births in 1946 considered the costs in some detail. It showed the expenses of maternity care and the difficulties these posed for poorer families in the era immediately before the start of the NHS.[33] Unfortunately, corresponding information has not been collected in such detail in more recent surveys. Most of what follows has therefore been taken from Miranda Mugford's review.[235]

Measuring costs of maternity care

As we described earlier, falling numbers of births and shortening lengths of postnatal stay in the early 1970s led to spare capacity in consultant hospitals. The requirement to fill beds and maintain 'efficiency' was achieved by increasing the proportion of births taking place in such units. As a result, occupancy in GP maternity units fell, and average costs per case increased as the fixed costs of the units were divided among the falling number of women delivering in them.

The words 'efficiency' and 'cost-effectiveness' are often used very loosely to imply that a service could be provided at lower cost. They convey the impression, however, that a formal economic appraisal of alternative ways of organising care has been carried out. An economic appraisal starts by defining the aims of the service, and continues by enumerating and measuring the costs and consequences of different options for meeting those aims. The emphasis of NHS maternity service planning has understandably been on minimising maternal and perinatal mortality. In recent years, although this aim still dominates, the comfort and wishes of childbearing women have been included as explicit policy objectives.[65]

Resources for maternity care may be provided from many sources, as shown in Table 13. In measuring the costs of care, health service planning concentrates on the resources paid for by district health authorities. Thus costs borne by families, and costs falling to other agencies, such as family health services authorities or local authority departments of social services, may not be considered.

Table 13

Measuring the full costs of maternity care

Whose resources?	Examples

Public purse

NHS purchasers of health services (district health authorities)	Contracts with providers of maternity services.
Providers of NHS maternity services	
NHS trusts, directly managed units	Hospital bed use, clinic use, home visits, ambulances.
General practitioners	Maternity medical services.
Social services	Social workers, home helps.
Social security	Benefits and other payments.

Family costs

Travel, extra help with domestic work, lost income.

Voluntary agencies

Charities supporting local hospitals	Equipment, amenities.
Voluntary support groups	Childbirth preparation, postnatal support, hospital voluntary work.

Even within the NHS district, there may be more than one provider unit and within each of these, services used for maternity care may fall under several budget headings. For example, costs of hospital administration, laboratories, pharmacy and medical salaries are not usually the responsibility of the midwifery manager. The apparently 'optimal' solution may differ, depending upon the viewpoint from which the maternity services are evaluated. Where costs and convenience to the users of the services are excluded from the cost-effectiveness equation by health service managers, the objectives of the service are unlikely to be achieved.

Economies of scale in NHS hospitals

In economic theory, organisations increase in their efficiency in terms of average cost per unit of output as they grow larger, because fixed costs are spread over a larger number of output units. Accounting data from the NHS are only just beginning to be separately available for the maternity specialty, but average costs per in-patient day by hospital type have been published annually for some years. Hospitals with maternity units were only classified as maternity hospitals when at least 90 per cent of discharges are maternity cases. Such units are unusual, and it is more frequently the case that maternity units of any size are part of an acute hospital. An analysis of average daily in-patient costs in English acute hospitals of different sizes in the financial year ending 31 March 1986 looked separately at patient care costs and general costs. Larger hospitals had higher patient care costs but this may have been a consequence of a more complex caseload. When these direct care costs were excluded, the general running costs per patient per day were lower in the smaller units. Thus, there was no evidence of economies of scale in larger units.

Average costs can disguise important variations between the hospitals in which maternity units are situated. Comparison between the average cost per in-patient day for all patients in hospitals with 'isolated' GP maternity units and with those in hospitals with consultant obstetric units in two districts in Oxfordshire revealed wide variations in average costs. In the hospitals with 'isolated' GP maternity units, the highest average costs per in-patient day were still lower than the costs in hospitals with consultant obstetric units, however.

These hospital cost figures could be deceptive in two ways. Firstly, they are an average of all specialties and do not indicate the costs of providing for maternity in-patient care. Secondly, as average costs, they do not necessarily measure the extra, or incremental, amount that would be needed to care for additional patients. This figure could be lower or higher depending on the capacity of existing resources at the unit. Thus, in a unit with low occupancy and high average costs per case, the additional or marginal cost of taking in further patients might be very small.

Comparisons of costs of maternity care in different settings

Although NHS financial data do not give very much separate information about maternity care costs, research papers comparing costs of different types of care have been published.

Research in the early 1970's[236] compared costs of maternity care to the health service for women delivering in eight different settings: a city consultant unit, a city GP unit, four rural isolated GP units, home delivery in the city, and rural home delivery. The authors measured average costs rather than incremental costs, and divided costs between women receiving some intervention at delivery and others. Costs to GPs and the local authority, which at that time was the employer of community midwives, were included, but not costs met by families. The authors of the study found that, for women who had had no intervention at delivery, costs per case were lower in the consultant unit than for any of the GP units. Home delivery also cost less than GP unit delivery.

Later, in the mid 1970's, a study[237] compared average hospital costs for maternity care in consultant units and in GP units in a Scottish health board area. The authors observed that isolated GP units and the consultant unit had different cost structures. The GP units had higher overhead costs because of the relatively low occupancy, but lower direct treatment costs. They did not estimate

costs separately for deliveries of different complexities. Costs for
consultant unit deliveries were higher and the difference was most
noticeable when comparing the costs of care for the day of delivery.
These higher costs are partly explained by the concentration of
women with complications in consultant units.

When comparing the costs of separate elements of maternity care
at the different units the authors concluded that it would be a more
efficient use of resources if women who delivered in the consultant
unit were discharged to the GP units for most of their postnatal
stay. This is a policy which was adopted in many districts with
isolated GP units. The alternatives, in the absence of the GP units,
would be either longer stays in the consultant units, or early
discharge home.

In the late 1970's, John Stilwell compared costs of care for women
who had a booked home delivery with matched women who
delivered in a GP unit.[238] These costs were compared with
estimated costs of normal delivery in the consultant unit. Public
sector costs for care were lowest for home delivery. Care for
women who delivered in the GP maternity unit was less costly to
the public purse than consultant care. This study also measured
costs to the family, taking account of extra help and travel costs,
and found that these were lowest for GP unit deliveries.

Maternity care which is provided in small community or cottage
hospitals cannot be considered in isolation from the other functions
of those hospitals. The maternity unit shares administrative and
some staff costs with other users, including GP surgery, geriatrics,
or convalescent and respite care. Closure of one function may affect
the overall viability of the hospital within the community.

A further problem in economic evaluation is allowing for capital
costs in particular for the use and value of buildings. This was not
discussed in the maternity costing studies referred to earlier. A
comparison[239] of different ways of organising surgery in an NHS
district, either in small 'acute' hospitals, or in the central district
general hospital, did take account both of capital costs and costs to
service users.[238] The most favourable solution, taking account of
these costs, was to upgrade operating facilities in smaller units,
rather than to centralise all surgery in the district general hospital.
This option would not have been indicated by comparing NHS

hospital running costs alone. Although there are clearly differences between local surgery and GP maternity care, there are also important parallels in that both need equipment and space. Also, in both cases there is a need for arrangements for emergency cover and transfer, and for selection of an optimum and appropriate caseload.

Costings of care in different settings in Scotland, for a policy review published in 1993, took a different approach. Care was costed according to the woman's original booking.[240] Thus, for women booking for home or isolated GP units, assumptions about transfers to consultant care were built into the costings. The average costs of care were estimated as £1,407 for a woman booked for home birth, £1,446 for a 'domino' birth and £1,991 for a GP maternity unit. The estimated costs for women booking in consultant units was £1,661 for low-risk cases and £2,535 for high-risk cases. The estimated costs for booking in places other than an obstetrician-led unit are therefore very sensitive to assumptions about transfer rates.

The Expert Maternity Group, which was set up to review NHS policy on maternity care in England did not attempt to cost the changes it recommended, although there was an implicit assumption that no new money would be available.[241] One of the objectives set out in its report *Changing childbirth* was that 'the service provided must represent value for money and the costs and benefits of alternative arrangements assessed locally.'[241] The accompanying action point stated that 'purchasers should agree with providers a programme to review the use of current resources, with particular emphasis on reducing unnecessary duplication'.[241]

Closure of small units on economic grounds

The continuing closures of small units and centralisation of maternity care are not based on good evidence about the cost-effectiveness of this policy. There are few studies of costs in GP maternity units, and these all date from a decade or more ago. The cost-effectiveness of GP maternity care is, in any case, a relative concept, and requires comparative evidence about the cost-effectiveness of consultant obstetric care. This has yet to be studied in any detail.

Closures of small units on grounds of rationalisation may simply represent a transfer of costs between sectors of the economy, in particular from NHS to individual families or to social services and social security. Districts may lose unmeasured resources, as voluntary support for community hospitals may not be transferred to the district hospital on closure of the small units.

Methods of option appraisal or cost-effectiveness analysis do not seem to be used widely in maternity care planning. One reason for this is the difficulty in obtaining suitable NHS accounting data. This situation may improve if and when the recommendations of the Steering Group on Health Services Information and NHS initiatives for resource management are implemented. These will not provide data about costs borne by those using the health services, however. For this information, independent surveys continue to be necessary.

The costs of change

Similar arguments can apply to changes made for other reasons, notably those aimed at providing more continuity of care and carer. To assist the deliberations of the Expert Maternity Group, a consensus conference was held in March 1993. Its statement, published as Annex 4 of the Group's report, referred to the lack of data on resources and went on to say 'there are examples where choice does appear to be restricted by a lack of resources and levels of service and the facilities available in different areas vary considerably. But there is also some evidence that changes will bring about resource savings, such as the better use of professional skills, other changes, such as making delivery rooms more homely could be introduced without significant extra spending.'[241] Despite this, the statement went on to acknowledge that resources are needed to bring about change and recommended that the Government should 'provide pump-priming and transitional funds to facilitate a diverse range of care and the consequent training that will be needed to implement these changes.'[241]

Parents' views about the place of birth

As we have already pointed out, the degree to which parents in general, and mothers in particular, feel satisfied with their experience and the care they receive can and has been used in analyses comparing different places of birth. The rapid decline up to 1980 in the proportion of births at home and the subsequent low level, might be taken as an indication that women prefer to give birth in hospital. The available research findings suggest that the opposite may be true, however.

One of the first surveys to ask where women wanted to give birth was that undertaken by the Joint Committee of the Royal College of Obstetricians and Gynaecologists and the Population Investigation Committee in 1946. Just over 90 per cent of the 15,130 women who gave birth in the first week of March of that year were successfully interviewed about the 'Social and economic aspects of childbirth'.[33]

When asked about reasons for their choice of place of delivery, 50.2 per cent of those who gave birth at home claimed to have done so because it was their preferred location. In contrast, only 16.6 per cent of those giving birth in hospital indicated that this had been their preference. Unsuitable housing conditions was the reason most people gave for delivering in hospital. The authors of the study concluded, 'The general indication . . . is that many women would prefer a good domiciliary maternity service, provided that some domestic help was available and housing conditions were improved.'[33]

Regrettably, the subsequent national birth surveys in 1958 and 1970 tended to focus on medical rather than social and economic questions and so the 1946 survey is one of the very few sources of national data on this issue. Most of the subsequent research done to determine women's preferences about the place of birth has involved small, non-random groups of women and rather crude attempts at attitude measurement. In all of the surveys of women who have experienced both home and hospital delivery, the vast majority preferred home, however.[229,242-245]

A postal survey of a random sample of 2,400 births in England and Wales in 1975 found that 92 per cent of women who were delivered at home but had had their previous baby in hospital preferred the home delivery. Only 23 per cent of those who had their baby in hospital but the previous baby at home preferred hospital.[246]

These studies are also almost certainly subject to the selection biases which beset place of delivery analyses. Women who have had a previous delivery in hospital and found it unsatisfactory are more likely to opt for a home birth for subsequent deliveries than those women who were satisfied with their hospital deliveries. The same would apply to women having negative experiences when giving birth at home. Given the huge disparity in the absolute numbers of women giving birth at home and in hospital, however, the flow of disenchanted mothers is largely going to be from hospital to home. Thus, the population of women who gave birth at home may well contain a disproportionate number of women who were dissatisfied with hospital delivery.

A persistent feature of the debate on place of birth has been the assertion, often made in pejorative terms, that women wanting to maintain choice about where and how to give birth are just a vocal, middle class minority.[247-251] Certainly, recent campaigns for better maternity services have tended, like many other campaigns, to be dominated by middle class women but this does not mean that the views they promote are unrepresentative. Indeed the evidence suggests that their views are representative of other women.

A recent survey a women's views and experiences of birth in five hospitals in Edinburgh found that 80 per cent of middle class mothers were offered a choice of hospital compared with only 64 per cent of working class women. When it came to preferences for 'low technology' approaches to birth such as choosing a position for birth or remaining mobile during labour there were no differences according to class.[252] These findings echo those of a national survey of childbirth undertaken in 1975. This showed that while a higher proportion of middle class women felt they had been given a choice about whether their labour was induced, there were no social class differences when it came to wanting a choice.[253] The absence of social class differences has also been reported in other studies of preferences for place of birth.[254] A study of home births from a practice in North London, which gives the choice of a home birth to any woman the staff consider clinically appropriate, reported that working class women welcome being given the option.[178]

The most common explanation given by women for preferring home delivery was that it did not involve separation from their partner and other members of the family. Other reasons given included negative feelings about the quality of care in hospital obstetric units, but these were mentioned less often. The main reasons for preferring hospital deliveries were that they provided more rest and greater safety.[242,245,255,256]

With the majority of births taking place in consultant obstetric units, more recent research into parents' views on the place of birth has been largely confined to studying women's preferences rather than their actual experiences. This is problematic because, apart from those who have been dissatisfied, women tend to express a preference for whatever type of delivery they have had.[257] This, coupled with findings which show that a sizeable proportion of women feel that they are given little or no choice about where to give birth, means that survey questionnaires asking women to make hypothetical choices about places of birth which they have no experience may elicit responses which are difficult to interpret.

Such difficulties were highlighted by a postal survey of all 192 women who gave birth at home in Nottingham in 1980 and 1981.[255] Questionnaires were also sent to a random sample of 365 women who delivered in hospital during the same period. Ninety per cent of those who gave birth at home and 88 per cent of those delivered in hospital said they would choose the same location next time. It was noted, however, that there was considerable non-response to this question for reasons which the authors described as 'obscure'. It is quite probable that being asked where you want to give birth when the overwhelming majority of births take place in hospital, may seem irrelevant. Furthermore, women who were not planning another child may have felt the question did not apply to them.[257]

There still appears to be a considerable interest in home births in spite of the fact that in the last few decades only a very small minority of women have had a planned home delivery. In a study of a cohort of 1,000 consecutive births in one London maternity hospital, women were sent a questionnaire one year after delivery.[258] The researchers claimed that this 'large and representative group of mothers . . . spurned home delivery'. This is rather misleading because what the results actually showed was that just over half of the respondents actually disagreed with the statement 'Home births ought to be encouraged'. Sixteen per cent agreed with the statement and the remainder neither agreed or disagreed. In addition a survey based on women giving birth in one London teaching hospital, to which slightly less than two thirds responded, cannot be considered truly representative.

A very small proportion of women giving birth in Great Britain during the last decade have actually had a planned home birth. Consequently, as women no longer perceive home birth as an option, estimating likely demand, were such a choice to be more widely available, is difficult. As correspondence in the *British Medical Journal* in 1992 highlighted,[259] the vast majority of women now express a preference for hospital birth. Estimates suggest that somewhere between 5 and 15 per cent of women would opt for home birth given a free choice. Thus, although demand is quite small this would still represent some 30,000 to 90,000 births per annum, which is considerably more than the 9211 planned and unplanned births at home in 1992.

Where to be born?

Some conclusions

Our review of the evidence about 'Where to be born?' suggests the following conclusions:

1. There is no evidence to support the claim that the safest policy is for all women to give birth in hospital.

2. The statistical association between the increase in the proportion of hospital deliveries and the fall in the crude perinatal mortality rate seems unlikely to be explained either wholly or in part by a cause and effect relationship.

3. No satisfactory explanation has been found for the higher crude perinatal mortality rate observed for births occurring before the mid 1970s in hospitals with consultant obstetric facilities compared with those in other places.

4. Lack of data means that it is not possible to conclude, with any degree of confidence, that babies born to low risk women in hospitals with consultant obstetric facilities are exposed to a greater or lesser risk of death due to obstetric intervention than similar babies born elsewhere.

5. The rise between 1970 and 1980 in the crude perinatal mortality rate for births at home can almost certainly be explained by the disproportionate increase in the proportion of unplanned births at home relative to those planned to occur there, as a consequence of the fall in the overall number of home births.

6. The policy of closing small obstetric units on the grounds of safety or cost is not supported by the available evidence.

7. For women at low risk who give birth in hospital, there is no clear evidence of differences between the mortality and morbidity of babies born to women giving birth under the care of consultant obstetricians and those whose deliveries are supervised by general practitioners.

8. The poorer outcomes among women transferred from home or general practitioner units compared with women who were not transferred probably results from selective referral of women with problems. Although there is no conclusive evidence, it is likely that this selection process, rather than the adverse effects of obstetric intervention, accounts for high mortality rates in hospital, compared with planned births at home or in isolated general practitioner units.

9. There is some evidence, although not conclusive, that morbidity is higher among mothers and babies cared for in an institutional setting. For some women, it is possible but not proven, that the iatrogenic risk associated with institutional delivery may be greater than any benefit conferred.

10. The few studies of cost done in the United Kingdom have found no evidence that care in general practitioner maternity units is uneconomic for the public sector or its users. There is insufficient recent evidence from which to draw any conclusions about the cost of home births.

11. A majority of women who had experienced both home and hospital deliveries preferred to have their babies at home, although they are more likely to include a disproportionate number of women who had sought home delivery after a hospital delivery with which they had been dissatisfied.

The debate and the evidence

These conclusions run counter to most of the policy recommendations made during the early 1980s by the back bench House of Commons Social Services Committee,[63] the government[131] and the Maternity Services Advisory Committee.[65] In 1985, the government confirmed its view that a hospital with a consultant maternity unit was the safest place for all births. In a parliamentary debate on maternity units, John Patten, then the Under-secretary of State for Health said:

> By and large, it is the government's view, and it remains their view, that women should be encouraged to have babies in the larger and properly staffed units of district general hospitals, which can offer the whole range of obstetric, paediatric and supporting services necessary to cope with any emergencies at the time when the life of the infant is most frail and when the life of the mother may be threatened.[131]

Meanwhile these policies were being questioned in the light of the body of evidence which had accumulated and the debate about its interpretation. A meeting on 'Pregnancy care in the 1980s' held at the Royal Society of Medicine in 1980 included contributions from midwives, general practitioners and obstetricians and papers on statistics from Marjorie Tew and from Eva Alberman, who had been epidemiological advisor to the Peel Committee and the House of Commons Social Services Committee.[260]

The British Journal of Obstetrics and Gynaecology took up this theme in 1986 when it published a series of articles on place of birth.[99,101,157,261] Accompanying these was a leader written by Eva Alberman. In this she said:

> . . . all the available evidence suggests that in carefully selected and well-supervised low-risk deliveries the extra risk to the mother and baby attributable only to the absence of hospital facilities must be low, and the satisfaction of a successful delivery high. Against this must be set the chance of needing an emergency transfer during, or after the delivery . . . [262]

More recently, when giving evidence to the House of Commons Health Committee in 1991, she expressed respect for Marjorie Tew, whose work she said had made her think hard about her earlier assumptions. She said that 'It is extremely difficult statistically to prove that for a normal delivery home birth is any safer than hospital birth.'[263] and said of her position, 'I still sit on the fence.'[263]

The first edition of *Where to be born ? The debate and the evidence* was published in June 1987. Its conclusions, which were very similar to those in this more recent edition, did not appear to have any impact on the Department's policy at the time. Later that year, replying to a parliamentary question from Labour spokesperson Harriet Harman about plans for the maternity services, the Under-secretary of State for Health, Edwina Currie reiterated the government's existing policy:

> We aim to minimise the risks to babies by encouraging delivery in hospital preferably with access to the full range of facilities which are likely to be found only on district general hospital sites.[264]

The reply went on to claim that this policy was responsible for the fall in perinatal and maternal mortality since 1979. In 1989, a parliamentary question asking specifically about policies for rural maternity units, many of which do not have consultant obstetric facilities, elicited a similar response.[265]

This position was restated yet again in November 1991, when a parliamentary question asked whether the Department had 'issued any guidance superseding the advice in *Maternity care in action* that "every mother should be encouraged to have her baby in a maternity unit"'. Phrases used on many previous occasions were repeated in the reply:

> No. The Department's policy remains that, as unforeseen circumstances can occur in any birth, every mother should be encouraged to have her baby in a maternity unit where emergency facilities are readily available. However, women should be able to make an informed choice about where to have their baby and discuss the options available with their general practitioner, midwife and obstetrician.[266]

When asked by an opposition health spokesperson, Harriet Harman, what research it had funded on place of delivery and what were its conclusions, the Department replied by referring to our review article in the British Journal of Obstetrics and Gynaecology,[261] but did not quote its conclusions.

As we have observed elsewhere in this book, the organisations representing the professions involved in providing care during childbirth have taken different stances on policy about place of birth and had varying degrees of influence over the policy process.

The Royal College of Obstetricians and Gynaecologists (RCOG) has enjoyed considerable influence on national policy about place of birth. Recommendations made by the College have often reappeared in subsequent government policy statements. In the 1980s, many government pronouncements seem to have been derived from a report by the RCOG on antenatal and intrapartum care. This stated that:

> In the present state of knowledge it is not possible to predict with accuracy which labours will be uncomplicated. It is therefore hoped that few, if any, pregnant women will be delivered at home.[267]

This report also endorsed a recommendation made by a joint working party of the Royal College of General Practitioners (RCGP) and the RCOG that general practitioners should only deliver women who had been carefully selected, in facilities immediately adjacent to consultant obstetric units.[267] Similarly, a report published in 1988 by anaesthetists specialising in obstetric work recommended that deliveries should not take place in small units without anaesthetic facilities.[268]

Midwives conduct the majority of deliveries but until recently they have had far less influence than doctors on national policy about the place of birth. Organisations representing midwives have taken a rather different perspective from that expressed by the RCOG. Midwives' organisations have emphasised that informed choice, continuity of care and adequate support are issues which need to be taken as seriously as safety. In a joint statement issued in 1983, the Royal College of Midwives (RCM) and the Health Visitors' Association said:

> The midwife should ensure that each pregnant woman is enabled to make an informed choice about the place of confinement. At present this freedom of choice is regrettably curtailed. There are seldom sufficient midwives to allow for even a limited choice and home delivery is often inhibited by inadequate medical cover.[269]

In a later policy document published in 1987, the RCM also acknowledged that doubt existed 'about the assumption that the safest place for delivery of all women is the consultant unit'.[270]

Some general practitioners with a strong interest in maternity care have also challenged the policy of encouraging all women to give birth in hospitals with specialist obstetric units and the consequent loss of isolated maternity units many of which served rural communities. Following a conference on general practitioner obstetrics in Birmingham in 1989, they formed a group called the Association for General Practice Maternity Care.[191] This name did not reflect the multidisciplinary approach which the association has always advocated and the extent to which midwives also became members. It has since been renamed the Association for Community-based Maternity Care.

Thus, by the end of the 1980s very clear differences had emerged between the professional groups concerned about policy on place of birth. These differences were made explicit in a policy document entitled *Maternity care in the new NHS - a joint approach* issued by the three royal colleges. This acknowledged that:

> The three Colleges view the issue of the place of delivery from differing standpoints. The RCOG considers that the range of specialist skills can only be realistically provided if the District General Hospital is the normal place of delivery. The RCM believes that an increased number of births could take place at home to the satisfaction of mothers and with safety. The RCGP is concerned that in certain geographical circumstances the clinical advantages of DGH care are outweighed by the practical and social disadvantages of distance from home and that small general

practitioner units have a place in this respect.[271]

It could be said that these different positions are as much a reflection of each organisation's desire to protect its own territory as a concern to satisfy the needs and preferences of service users. Nevertheless, the positions also reflect different views of pregnancy and birth. Midwives are inclined to assume that this is a normal process unless and until complications are diagnosed. On the other hand doctors' training and role makes them more likely to focus on the risks of abnormality.

While the positions of the professional organisations were crystallising, groups representing the interests of service users continued to campaign for a more pluralistic pattern of maternity care which permitted real choice of place of birth. For example, the First International Conference on Home Birth was held in London in 1987. Its local organisers included the Association for Improvements in the Maternity Services, the Active Birth Movement and the Independent Midwives Association.

In 1990, the Maternity Alliance, an umbrella group whose member organisations include a variety of professional and lay bodies, organised a seminar in the House of Commons entitled 'Where to be born. Choice and safety in maternity care'. This was organised in response to a request by Roger Freeman, who was at that time Parliamentary Under-secretary of State for Health, and wished to hear the evidence about small maternity units. The audience included two other MPs, Audrey Wise and Sir Frank Price, both of whom were members of the House of Commons Social Services Committee. At the end of the seminar, Roger Freeman announced that on the basis of what he had heard, he would not approve any further closures of small maternity units. The choice was taken out of his hands, however. Less than two weeks later, he was moved to the Department of Transport.

The House of Commons Health Committee's enquiry

Some months later, the new House of Commons Health Committee, chaired by Nicholas Winterton and whose members included Audrey Wise, decided to launch an investigation into maternity services. In contrast to the three previous parliamentary investigations into maternity issues undertaken by its predecessor, the emphasis this time was on care in uncomplicated pregnancy and birth, rather than on perinatal and infant mortality.

When Virginia Bottomley, then Minister for Health, first gave evidence to the Health Committee she gave no indication of any change in the Department's policy on place of birth.[272] The second time she gave evidence, she was referred to the parliamentary question about research on place of delivery and asked explicitly how the Department had used the research it had funded. In her response on this occasion, there was a hint of a slight change in position. She said:

I was trying to make clear to the Committee that there is no overwhelming evidence, unequivocal evidence about the relative merits of different settings and some of the evidence is conflicting in some ways.[273]

The Committee referred to this in its report entitled *Maternity services*, which was published in March 1992.[274] Its first two conclusions were radically different from those of its predecessor, the Social Services Committee:

On the basis of what we have heard, this Committee must draw the conclusion that the policy of encouraging all women to give birth in hospital cannot be justified on the grounds of safety.

and

Given the absence of conclusive evidence, it is no longer acceptable that the pattern of maternity care provision should be driven by presumptions about the applicability of a medical model of care based on unproven assertions.[274]

The Health Committee's report was wide ranging and also included recommendations about subjects such as neonatal care and long term follow up of babies who received it, care for women from minority ethnic groups and women with disabilities and on maternity benefits. Much of the press coverage focused on the recommendations about place of birth, however. These tended to be somewhat misrepresented as suggesting that 'MPs want more women to give birth at home'.[275] Media coverage also highlighted the strong emphasis placed on the importance of the role of midwives in providing care for women who have normal deliveries with headlines such as 'MPs back more home births with midwives in charge.'[276] In contrast, the recommendations for changes to maternity benefits were largely ignored.

The Winterton Report, as the Health Committee's report has now come to be known, appears to signal a significant shift in thinking at the highest levels of public representation, although it had not at this point affected government policy. The Committee said in its report 'We have placed women at the centre of this enquiry and report.'[274] It undoubtedly took greater account of the views of women than earlier parliamentary reports. The views of professional groups, in particular those of the RCOG, are far less prominent than in earlier reports. This is particularly noticeable when it comes to the discussions and recommendations on place of birth.

The RCOG's opposition to the Health Committee's report was considerable. The College organised a press conference on the day when the report was published, in order to criticise it. In its subsequent more detailed response to the report, the RCOG voiced concern about the recommendations on place of birth. The College stated that it 'rejects the view that national policy of encouraging all women to deliver in hospital can now be abandoned and maintains its policy that hospital delivery maximises safety for mothers and babies.'[277] There is also a hint of 'shroud waving' in the College's response, that accepts that there may be alternatives but is of the view that 'major changes should not be implemented without considering their effects on maternal and perinatal mortality and morbidity.'[277]

When the government replied to the Committee in July 1992, its response was not markedly different from its earlier position:

The safety of mother and child must be the prime consideration.

It is impossible to predict all the problems which may arise in labour. Women have therefore been encouraged to give birth in hospital where back-up facilities are available in an emergency but the Government recognises that there are women for whom home birth may be an option they would prefer. Health authorities are obliged to recognise a woman's right to choose, and see that a midwifery service is available for a woman to give birth at home, if that is her choice.[278]

The government responded to the many other issues covered by the Committee's report by stating that:

The measures which have been introduced through the Government's NHS and community care reforms, and the Patient's Charter initiatives will enhance the quality and responsiveness of all health care services, not just the maternity services.[278]

It listed no less than nine enquiries, committees and other initiatives which were 'aimed at ensuring other further improvements in maternity services'. In addition it mentioned that the Maternity Unit Study Team was expected to report shortly and would give examples of good practice in units run by GPs or midwives.

The reference to the 'NHS and Community Care reforms' in the government's response serves as a reminder that this most recent episode in the debate on place of birth was taking place at a time when there was a general trend within the NHS to move care out of hospital. This means that the move to community-based maternity care coincides with policy developments such as greater use of day surgery, shorter stays in hospital and closing large long stay hospitals for people with mental illnesses or learning difficulties and moving residents into a variety of community settings. Earlier hopes that adequate community care might be cheaper than hospital care have proved unfounded and the adequacy of some of the care provided in the community has been called into question.[279] Thus, just as in the earlier part of this century changes in policy about maternity care were influenced by and formed part of a more general tendency to move care into hospitals, changes in maternity policies at the end of the century seem to form part of a general movement away from hospital care.

The government's reply to the Health Committee also announced that it was establishing an expert committee to review policy on care during childbirth and to make recommendations. This became known as the Expert Maternity Group and was chaired by Baroness Cumberlege, the Parliamentary Under-secretary of State (Lords).

The Maternity Unit Study Team's report, published in January 1993, set out 'broad principles' based on visits to six units. These included both decentralised 'isolated' units distant from a district general hospital consultant maternity unit, and midwife-led and GP-led services located within consultant maternity units. It did not review the evidence and referred instead to the government's 'belief that consultant-led units in district general hospitals provide the safest setting for care.' Nevertheless, it went on to acknowledge that universal application of this policy was neither practicable or acceptable particularly in areas with dispersed populations.[280]

Changing childbirth

The Expert Maternity Group's report [241] *Changing childbirth* was published in August 1993. Like the Winterton Report it signalled a considerable change in the direction of policy for maternity care. It also stressed that the service must be 'woman centred'. To achieve this, it recommended that midwives should have a more prominent role, with every pregnant woman having a named midwife even if her care is led by a GP or obstetrician. Increasing choice is a key theme of the report, with recommendations that each woman should be provided with accurate and unbiased information about the options available so that she can make informed decisions, for instance about where she receives that care.

In discussing place of birth the report commented that:

Whether a mother with an uncomplicated pregnancy is putting herself and her child at any greater risk by choosing to have her baby away from a general hospital is a topic that has been argued with vehemence and emotion for decades. The inability to reach agreement after this length of time suggests there is no clear answer. The job of midwives and doctors, therefore, must be to provide the woman with as accurate and objective information as possible, whilst avoiding personal bias or preference.[241]

A survey commissioned by the Expert Maternity Group from MORI Health Research asked 1005 women who had given birth since 1989 whether they would like to have the option of another type of care and delivery if they became pregnant again. Seventy two per cent said they would have liked an option other than delivery in a consultant unit. Of these, 22 per cent said they would have liked the choice of a home birth and 44 per cent a 'domino' delivery. These accounted for 16 per cent and 32 per cent of all women questioned, respectively.[241]

Each section of *Changing childbirth* contained one or more 'action points' for implementing its proposals. A closing section entitled 'Action for change' listed ten indicators of success to be achieved within five years. It proposed that every woman should have and know a 'lead professional' and a named midwife. At least 30 per cent should have a midwife as the 'lead professional'. Midwives should have direct access to some beds in all maternity units. At least 30 per cent of women should be admitted under the management of a midwife and at least 75 per cent should know the person who cares for them during delivery. It calls for the numbers of antenatal visits to be reviewed and for all ambulances to have a paramedic able to support midwives transferring women from home to hospital during delivery. Finally, all women should be entitled to carry their own case notes and have access to information about local services.

Predictably the report has had a mixed response. It has been welcomed by the RCM and groups representing users of the maternity services.[281,282] The RCM's official response, which welcomed the report enthusiastically, was largely devoted to discussing how to take its proposals forward. It did so under the headings of information and communication, management of change, education, audit and legislative change.[283] In a much briefer response, the Royal College of GPs welcomed the report by acknowledging the role of midwives in normal maternity care while stressing the need for them to work with the GPs who have responsibility for longer term care of the families concerned.[284]

On the other hand, the British Medical Association[285] and the RCOG[286] have both expressed concern about the likely increase in the number of home births and the suggestion, in the report, that all women should be seen by a midwife but not necessarily by a doctor. It seems likely that it was in response to pressure from the RCOG that the report was issued as a consultative document rather than the policy document previously announced.[286]

Nevertheless, the College's response to the consultation on *Changing childbirth* showed some acknowledgment of a shift in policy although its overall message was unclear.[287] For example, it expressed the view that 'Much of this report is helpful . . .' Next it voiced concern that some of the suggestions for change had not been scientifically tested and called for more money for audit. It expressed support for the role of midwives as independent practitioners while also making the case for obstetricians and general practitioners having a role in 'normal obstetrics'. While acknowledging that women had a right to choose a home birth, it urged the Department of Health not to encourage home births at the moment and instead to seek evidence that they are not in any way less safe than those in hospital'.[287] This mixed message was also apparent in a pamphlet for parents on 'home births' written by the President of the College.[288] This gave advice on how to plan a home birth but devoted rather more space to advocating alternatives.

Although *Changing childbirth* was discussed throughout the United Kingdom, strictly it only applied to policy in England. The conclusion of the Scottish policy review document issued a few months earlier offered little encouragement for a shift to delivery outside hospital, but did advocate a greater use of 'Domino' deliveries and midwife-led units.[240] Slightly earlier in 1992, the *Protocol for investment in health gain*, issued by the Welsh Office, emphasised the need for women to have more control and an informed choice about the care given during pregnancy and childbirth.[289]

After the consultation period, the Department of Health

announced its acceptance of *Changing childbirth* in January 1994 with a press release entitled 'Women will have greater say in maternity care: mother and baby come first'.[290] At the same time health authorities were sent an 'Executive letter', entitled *Woman-centred maternity services*.[291] This instructed them to ensure that the recommendations of *Changing childbirth* were reflected in their 3-5 year purchasing strategies and their 1995/96 purchasing plans. It also announced an advisory group which was set up to support the NHS Executive in the implementation of *Changing childbirth*[292] and a Patient's Charter leaflet.[293]

This was launched by Baroness Cumberlege when speaking at a National Childbirth Trust Conference. Included in the information to which women should have access, is 'Where you can give birth (including at home)'.[293] The leaflet also said that health authorities should arrange to make it possible for women to go directly to a midwife for care. The accompanying press release stated more explicitly that 'you have the right to choose where your baby is born - in hospital or at home'[294] Both also responded to doctors' concerns by stating that women should have the opportunity to see a consultant obstetrician at least once during their pregnancy and, if problems were anticipated, a consultant paediatrician. Both the leaflet and the 'Executive letter' listed the ten indicators of success from *Changing childbirth*.

Signs of changing views could be seen in the *Report on confidential enquiries into maternal deaths* for the year 1988-90.[295] This was published early in 1994, and like the reports published in the 1980s, it contained no explicit analysis by place of delivery. Nevertheless, in reporting on the increasing numbers of deaths attributed to antepartum and postpartum haemorrhage, it said:

> The place of isolated units and GP units is still a subject of discussion. If death from haemorrhage occurs once in 100,000 deliveries a GP unit may encounter such a tragedy less than once in a century. In this triennium no death from postpartum haemorrhage occurred in a healthy woman who had a spontaneous vaginal delivery, and the key to maintaining safety in GP units is rigorous exclusion of women with risk factors.[120]

The report's overall recommendations included a section on 'domiciliary care'. This recommended that 'Adequate care in the community must be ensured for those mothers with special needs who are unable or unwilling to comply with professional advice'.[120] It went on to refer to the needs for adequate training for ambulance service paramedics, acknowledging that they, rather than obstetric flying squads are increasingly providing the care needed when acute obstetric emergencies occur outside hospital.

While it will undoubtedly continue, further debate on place of birth is likely to be somewhat sterile. There are two main reasons for this. Firstly, for women whose chances of adverse outcome are not very high, any differences between mortality rates associated with different places of birth are now likely to be very small. As a result, such differences may have little impact on such women's choice to give birth in places other than hospitals with consultant units. Secondly, it seems clear that whatever the evidence, many leading obstetricians are unlikely to move away from their position of advocating hospital delivery for all women. The RCOG argues that the evidence is equivocal and that more research is needed, particularly on home births, before policy can be changed.

Although general practitioners may play a smaller part in providing maternity care than in the past, they still have a crucial role in ensuing that women have a choice. In time, women may come to see midwives as their first point of contact with the maternity services but at present most women start by approaching their general practitioner. It is essential therefore to ensure that GPs have a positive view of the range of choices available.

It is too early to assess the full impact of recent changes to the NHS, including the introduction of the internal market and, in particular, the purchaser provider split. This could potentially result in more diversity in the forms of maternity care available and thus give greater choice. Health authorities may gradually move away from purchasing maternity care on the basis of historic demands and patterns of referral and attempt to base purchasing on a detailed assessment of comparative costs, accessibility, and parents' choice as well as on safety and the availability of back up. On the other hand, the range of choices available may be restricted by financial constraints.

Changing childbirth has also been criticised from a different perspective, for taking a consumerist approach and satisfying the demands of middle class women while ignoring the concerns of women whose children are born into poor circumstances.[296] It is true that *Changing childbirth* made no response to the recommendations in the Winterton report about benefits and the financial needs of parents living in poverty. The remit of the Expert Maternity Group did not extend beyond NHS care and the fact that financial questions were not considered was acknowledged in the introduction to its report.

These pressing issues remain unanswered, however. Despite continued reminders from the Maternity Alliance and others that the proportion of all children who are born into families on means tested benefits rose from 21 per cent in 1988-89 to 30 per cent in 1992-93,[297] there has been no response in other areas of government policy. The government's reply to the Winterton report simply quoted existing benefit levels and arrangements, and reiterated its view that these were adequate.[278]

Nevertheless, there are no grounds for assuming that the middle class women who have the time and political skills to make their views known are unusual in wanting a choice about where and how to give birth.[298] Indeed, sensitivity to the way choices in maternity care relate to their wider financial circumstances and social needs should be an integral part of giving 'woman-centred' care to all women, but particularly those who are disadvantaged. Some specific ways of doing this were given in a code of practice published in June 1994 by the Commission for Racial Equality,[299]

We find ourselves completing this second edition of *Where to be born?* in a rather different climate from the one which prevailed when we finished the first edition. That edition ended with the rather depressing comment that 'the most striking feature of the debate about where to be born, however, is the way policy has been formed with very little reference to the evidence.' The Winterton report and *Changing childbirth* have both produced policy recommendations which do take account of the evidence available. Both stress the importance of demonstrating the effectiveness of all new forms of maternity care and their acceptability to the women for whom it is provided.

The change in policy may also reflect the increasing extent to which women's views are heard on the political stage. In recent years women have had a growing role in political parties at all levels and in formulating their health policy, in particular. In parliament, Labour back-bencher Audrey Wise drew on her own and other women's experiences in the key role she played in setting the agenda for the House of Commons Health Committee's report. Conservative minister Baroness Cumberlege did likewise when chairing the Expert Maternity Group and transforming many of the Committee's recommendations into policy. In the late 1980s, Conservative minister Edwina Currie and Labour shadow minister Harriet Harman drew on their own differing experiences when influencing their respective parties' policies. As we go to press Virginia Bottomley is Secretary of State for Health and two other women, Dawn Primarolo and Liz Lynne, are respectively Labour and Liberal Democrat spokespeople on health, with briefs which include maternity policy.

As a result of this greater emphasis on both effectiveness and women's views, we close this second edition in a much more optimistic mood than we did the first. Nevertheless, there is still cause for concern about a key aspect of information about maternity care. This is the routine data collection systems which are essential to monitor the activities of maternity services and the extent to which new policies do have the effect of changing childbirth. Of the four countries of the United Kingdom, only Scotland has a national data collection system which can produce reliable estimates of even such basic measures as caesarean section, instrumental delivery and induction rates. In England, Wales and Northern Ireland it is still the case, as Florence Nightingale wrote in 1871, 'that midwifery statistics are in an unsatisfactory condition'.[4] Her list of gaps in the information needed has a contemporary ring, at national level at least.

Such are the general sanitary state of hospitals, wards, houses and rooms where deliveries take place; the management adopted; the classes of patients; their state of health; the time they are kept in midwifery wards before and after delivery. These elements are directly connected with the questions at issue and yet our information is by no means full as we would wish - indeed is almost nothing.[4]

It is disappointing that with computing technology which would have been beyond her wildest dreams, so little has been achieved at national level, despite local developments in some places. Harnessing it to provide a useful description of what is happening in the maternity services is a challenge for the immediate future. Simply monitoring the ten 'indicators of success' set out in *Changing childbirth* and the subsequent 'Executive letter'[291] will not be sufficient.

Florence Nightingale's response to her lack of data was:

. . . our only resource at present is to deal with such statistical information as we possess and to ascertain fairly what it tells us . . .[4]

In this review, we have tried to follow this principle. We hope this will prove useful in making decisions about where to be born.

Glossary of terms

Abortion	death or expulsion of the fetus either spontaneously or by intention before 24 completed weeks of pregnancy. In addition, a pregnancy deliberately ended on grounds of fetal abnormality at any gestation is an abortion.
Alongside general practioner maternity unit	a general practitioner maternity unit which is on the same site as a consultant obstetric unit but is functionally separate with its own wards and delivery area.
Anaesthesia	a state in which the whole body (general anaesthesia) or part of it (local or regional anaesthesia) is insensible to pain.
Analgesia	lessening or abolition of sensation to pain or stimuli - may be general or local.
Antenatal	before the birth
Antepartum	before the onset of labour.
Booking for delivery	appropriate medical and midwifery services are booked for the time around the expected date of delivery - usually classified in terms of the intended place of delivery and type of care provided, for example, a GP bed in a consultant unit.
Congenital	existing at the time of birth.
Consultant obstetric maternity unit	a maternity unit in which women book with a consultant obstetrician to deliver under the supervision of midwives and obstetricians.

Epidural	a local anaesthetic injected around the spinal sac causing loss of sensation to the lower part of the body.
Episiotomy	surgical cut in perineum performed at the end of labour immediately before a vaginal birth.
Flying squad	an ambulance which is sent out from a consultant obstetric unit with specialist obstetric and paediatric staff and equipment to provide emergency care for a mother or baby in the community.
Fetal distress	signs from observations of the condition of the fetus which might indicate a potentially harmful environment in the womb. The most commons signs are abnormalities of fetal heart rate and rhythm and, in a cephalic presentation, meconium staining of the liquor.
General practitioner maternity unit	a maternity unit in which women book with a general practitiner to deliver under the supervision of midwives and general practitioners.
Gestation	pregnancy. Its duration is usually measured from the first day of the last menstrual period.
Gravidity	the total number of previous pregnancies, including those ending in miscarriage or abortion.
Haemorrhage	excessive bleeding. Usually refers to extreme loss of blood, or bleeding causing further internal or external damage.
Iatrogenic	caused by the process of diagnosis or treatment.
Induced abortion	abortion brought on purposefully using drugs or other means.
Induction of labour or abortion	Process by which uterine contractions are initiated artificially, either by breaking the membraneous sac around the baby or by drugs or both.
Integrated general practitioner maternity unit	a general practitioner maternity unit which shares common wards and delivery areas with a consultant obstetric unit.

Intended place of delivery	the planned place of delivery. Defined either as the place booked for delivery or the place intended immediately before the onset of labour.
Intrapartum	during labour.
Intrauterine	inside the uterus or womb.
Isolated general practitioner maternity unit	a general practitioner maternity unit which is geographically separated from the nearest consultant obstetric unit.
Live birth	a child which, after expulsion from the uterus at any gestation has breathed or shown any other sign of life, such as the beating of the heart, pulsation of the umbilical cord, or definite movement of voluntary muscles is considered as live born for legal and statistical purposes.
Midwife	person qualified to take responsibility for care during uncomplicated pregnancies and deliveries.
Midwife-led maternity care	a scheme or maternity unit in which women book with midwives for delivery under the supervision of midwives.
Miscarriage	the expulsion of a dead fetus, other than by intention, before the 24th week of completed pregnancy.
Morbidity	disease, abnormality.
Neonatal death	death within 28 days of live birth.
Neonatology	the medical specialty concerned with the care of ill newborn babies.
Obstetrics	the medical and surgical specialty concerned with (problems arising in) pregnancy, delivery and the puerperium.
Paediatrics	medical specialty concerned with the care of babies and children.

Parity	total number of previous live births and stillbirths. This does not include abortions or miscarriages.
Perinatal	around the birth. The number of stillbirths plus the number of deaths occurring less than one week after live birth expressed as a rate per thousand live and stillbirths is known as the perinatal mortality rate.
Perineum	area of pelvic floor between vagina and anus.
Postnatal	after birth, usually taken as a period of six weeks.
Post-partum	after delivery.
Puerperium	period after delivery during which the mother's body adjusts to the end of pregnancy.
Spontaneous abortion	miscarriage
Stillbirth	a baby which is born dead after 24 completed weeks of pregnancy. The legal definition is 'a child which has issued forth from its mother after 24 or more completed week of pregnancy and which did not at any time after being completely expelled from its mother breathe or show any signs of life'. Before October 1 1992, the word stillbirth applied to such events occurring after 28 or more completed weeks of pregnancy.
Termination of pregnancy	a pregnancy which is deliberately ended legally or illegally.
Uterus	womb

Sources of advice and information about maternity services

This contains firstly information about organisations with a particular focus on maternity care and secondly about organisations whose interests include maternity care. A third section contains details of organisations who represent people who provide maternity care. In drawing up this list we have made considerable use of the Patients' Association *Health address book* which contains useful information about a wide range of organisations. The following organisations should be able to help with information about maternity services in general. Some can also help with choices about place of birth with other particular aspects of maternity care:

National Childbirth Trust
Alexandra House
Oldham Terrace
Acton
London W3 6NH

0181 992 8637

National organisation with many local groups. Aims to offer information and support in pregnancy, childbirth and early parenthood and to help every parent make informed choices.

Maternity Alliance
15 Britannia Street
London WC1X 9JP

0171 837 1265

National organisation which can provide up to date information on a wide range of maternity issues including employment rights and maternity benefits.

Association for Improvements in the Maternity Services (AIMS)
40 Kingswood Avenue
London NW6 6LS

0181 960 5585

40 Leamington Terrace
Edinburgh EH10 4JL

0131 229 6259

Voluntary pressure group with some local groups. Offers support and advice about parents' rights, complaints procedures and choices within maternity care including home birth.

Twins and Multiple Births Association (TAMBA)
PO Box 30
Little Sutton
South Wirral L66 1TH

0151 348 0020 6.00 pm - 11.00 pm weekdays 10.00 am - 11.00 pm weekends
TAMBA Twinline 0732 868000

Self help organisation to encourage and support parents of twins, triplets or more.

Active Birth Centre
55 Dartmouth Park
London NW5 1SL

0171 267 3006

Runs antenatal workshops, yoga-based exercise classes, post-natal support groups, baby-relax classes, active birth teachers' courses and courses for couples.

Association for Community-based Maternity Care
Barn Croft
Temple Sowerby
Nr Penrith
Cumbria CA10 1RZ

017683 61232
017683 61980 (fax)

A group largely composed of professionals with lay input set up to foster maternity care in the community and in particular choice of place of birth.

Miscarriage Association
c/o Clayton Hospital
Wakefield
West Yorkshire WF1 3JS

01924 200799 Helpline (Answering machine outside office hours)
01924 200795

Gives support and information to women who have had a miscarriage

Support Around Termination for Fetal Abnormality (SAFTA)
29-30 Soho Square
London W1V 6JB

0171 439 6124 Helpline
0171 287 3753

Helps parents who discover that their baby is abnormal

Stillbirth and Neonatal Death Society (SANDS)
28 Portland Place
London W1N 4DE

0171 436 5881 Helpline
0171 436 7940

A national self-help organisation which offers support when a baby dies during pregnancy or around the time of birth.

The following organisations should be able to provide information about maternity services as part of their work of providing information about health services in general:

Community health councils	England and Wales
Local health councils	Scotland
Local health and social services councils	Northern Ireland

These local bodies are there to represent the interests of users of the NHS. They can give advice on local NHS services and entitlements. They should be able to help if you are having difficulties or wish to make a complaint. Look for them in your local phone directory or ask in your public library.

College of Health
St Margaret House
21 Old Ford Road
London E2 9PL

0181 983 1225

Aims to give people the information they need to make the most effective use of the NHS.

Health Service Commissioner
Church House
Great Smith Street
London SW1P 3PW

0171 276 2035

Investigates complaints against NHS authorities, including maladministration and failure to provide a service, but not clinical judgement. Complaints must be made in writing.

The Patients' Association
18 Victoria Park Square
Bethnal Green
London E2 9PF

0181 981 5676/5695

Represents patients' interests to government and professional bodies and all organisations involved in health matters.

Health Information Service

0800 665544

Provides information about the Patient's Charter, including the Maternity Charter.

Organisations who represent the professionals who provide maternity care

Royal College of General Practitioners
14 Princes Gate
London SW7 1PU

0171 581 6523

Royal College of Midwives
15 Mansfield Street
London W1M OBE

0171 580 6523

Royal College of Obstetricians and Gynaecologists
27 Sussex Place
London NW1 4RG

0171 262 5425

Association of Radical Midwives
62 Greetby Hill,
Ormskirk,
Lancs L39 2DT

01695 572776

References

1. Cochrane AL. Effectiveness and efficiency: random reflections on the Health Service. London: Nuffield Provincial Hospitals Trust, 1972.

2. Smith FB. The people's health 1830-1910. London: Croom Helm, 1979.

3. Donnison J. Midwives and medical men. New York: Schocken Books, 1977.

4. Nightingale F. Notes on lying-in institutions, together with a proposal for organising an institution for training midwives and midwifery nurses. London: Longmans, Green and Co., 1871.

5. Campbell R. Home births survey. Perinatal mortality by intended place of delivery for births occuring at home. England and Wales, 1979. PhD Thesis. London University, 1986. Unpublished.

6. Medline. US National Library of Medicine database.

7. BIDS. Bath University Interactive Data Services.

8. Loudon I. Deaths in childbed from the eighteenth century to 1935. Medical History 1986; 30:1-41.

9. Loudon I. Death in childbirth. An international study of maternal care and maternal mortality, 1800-1950. Oxford University Press, 1992.

10. General Register Office. Fifth annual report of the Registrar General for 1841. London: Longman, Brown, Green and Longman, 1843.

11. Pall Mall Gazette. Workhouse death rate in childbirth. Reproduced in: Journal of the Royal Statistical Society 1867; 30: 171-172.

12. Select Committee on Midwives Registration. Report. Parliamentary Papers 1892; IV.

13. Webb S, Webb B, eds. The break-up of the Poor Law, being part one of the Minority Report of the Poor Law Commission. London: Longman, Green and Co., 1909.

14. Newsholme A. Memorandum on health visiting and on maternity and child welfare centres. In: Supplement to the forty-fourth annual report of the Local Government Board 1914-15. Cd 8153. London: HMSO, 1916.

15. Local Government Board. Maternity and child welfare. Report on the provision made by Local Authorities in England and Wales. London: HMSO, 1917.

16. Local Government Board. Forty-eighth annual report. Supplement containing the report of the Medical Department for 1918-19. Cmd 462. London: HMSO, 1919.

17. Barnes J. Happier birthdays. The story of the National Birthday Trust. Sixth Rhys Williams Memorial lecture. Midwives Chronicle 1970; 83:406-411.

18. Williams S. The history of the National Birthday Trust Fund. Volume 1. In preparation.

19. Munro AE. Deaths in childbed. London: Smith, Elder & Co, 1879.

20. Williams W. Deaths in childbed, a preventable mortality. London: HK Lewis, 1904.

21. General Register Office. Thirty-third report of the Registrar General for 1870. London: HMSO, 1872.

22. Local Government Board. Forty-seventh annual report of the Local Government Board, 1917-18. Part I. Cd 9157. London: HMSO, 1918.

23. Ministry of Health. Annual report of the Chief Medical Officer, 1919-20. London: HMSO, 1920.

24. Ministry of Health. Memorandum with regard to maternity homes and hospitals. 15/MCW. London: HMSO, 1920.

25.   Campbell JM. Maternal mortality. Reports on public health and medical subjects no. 25. London: HMSO, 1924.

26.   Bonney V. An address (in abridged form) on the continued high maternal mortality of childbearing. The reason and the remedy. Lancet 1919; i:775-6.

27.   Campbell JM. The protection of motherhood. Reports on public health and medical subjects no. 48. London: HMSO, 1927.

28.   Macfarlane AJ. Statistics and policy making in the maternity services. Midwifery 1985; 1:150-161.

29.   Peretz E. A maternity service for England and Wales: local authority maternity care in the inter-war period in Oxford and Tottenham. In: Garcia J, Kilpatrick R, Richards M, eds. The politics of maternity care. Oxford: Clarendon Press, 1990.

30.   Registrar General's statistical review for the year 1927. London: HMSO, 1929.

31.   Registrar General's statistical review for the year 1932. London: HMSO, 1935.

32.   Registrar General's statistical review for the year 1937. London: HMSO, 1940.

33.   Royal College of Obstetricians and Gynaecologists, Population Investigation Committee. Maternity in Great Britain. Oxford: Oxford University Press, 1948.

34.   Macfarlane A, Mugford M. Birth counts: statistics of pregnancy and childbirth. London: HMSO, 1984.

35.   Office of Population Censuses and Surveys. Birth statistics, Series FM1. London: HMSO. Published annually.

36.   Lewis J. Mothers and maternity policies in the twentieth century. In: Garcia J, Kilpatrick R, Richards M, eds. The politics of maternity care. Oxford: Clarendon Press, 1990.

37.   Beinart J. Obstetric analgesia and the control of childbirth in twentieth century Britain. In: Garcia J, Kilpatrick R, Richards M, eds. The politics of maternity care. Oxford: Clarendon Press, 1990.

38. British Medical Association. The BMA and maternity services. British Medical Journal 1936; 1:656.

39. Oakley A. The trap of medicalised motherhood. New Society 1975; 34:639-641.

40. Comaroff J. Conflicting paradigms of pregnancy: managing ambiguity in antenatal encounter. In: Davis A, Horobin G, eds. Medical encounters. Experience of illness and treatment. London: Croom Helm, 1977.

41. Schwarz EW. The engineering of childbirth. In: Garcia J, Kilpatrick R, Richards M, eds. The politics of maternity care. Oxford: Clarendon Press, 1990.

42. British College of Obstetricians and Gynaecologists. Outline of a scheme for a national maternity service. London: BCOG, 1936.

43. Royal College of Obstetricians and Gynaecologists. Report on a national maternity service. London: RCOG, 1944.

44. Royal College of Obstetricians and Gynaecologists. Report on the obstetric service under the NHS. London: RCOG, 1954.

45. Webster C. The health services since the War. Volume I. Problems of health care, the National Health Service before 1957. London: HMSO, 1988.

46. Titmuss R. History of the Second World War. Problems of social policy. London: HMSO and Longmans, Green and Co., 1950.

47. Rhys Williams J. Letter to Harold Macmillan, 16 July 1954. MH 94254/2/19.

48. Butler NR, Bonham DG. Perinatal mortality. The first report on the 1958 British Perinatal Mortality Survey. Edinburgh and London: E & S Livingstone, 1963.

49. Ministry of Health. Report of the Maternity Services Committee (Chairman Lord Cranbrook). London: HMSO, 1959.

50. Ministry of Health. Report of the Ministry of Health for April 1950 to December 1951. Part I. Cmd 8655. London: HMSO, 1952.

51.   Standing Maternity and Midwifery Advisory Committee (Chairman, J. Peel). Domiciliary midwifery and maternity bed needs. London: HMSO, 1970.

52.   Heliman LM, Kohn SG, Palmer J. Early hospital discharge in obstetrics. Lancet 1962; i:227-232.

53.   Pinker GD, Fraser AC. Early discharge of maternity patients. British Medical Journal 1964; 2:99-100.

54.   Craig GA, Muirhead JMB. Obstetric aspects of the early discharge of maternity patients. British Medical Journal 1967; 3: 520-522.

55.   Arthurton MW, Bamford FN. Paediatric aspects of the early discharge of maternity patients. British Medical Journal 1967; 3:1351-1352.

56.   Sluglett J, Walker S. A general practitioner maternity unit. Lancet 1956; i:684-686.

57.   O'Sullivan V. General practitioner maternity beds in a large general hospital. British Medical Journal 1961; 2:1349-1350.

58.   Hobbs MST, Acheson ED. Perinatal mortality and the organisation of obstetric services in the Oxford Area in 1962. British Medical Journal 1966; 1:499.

59.   Department of Health and Social Security. Report of the Expert Group on Special Care for Babies (Chairman, W Sheldon). Reports on public health and medical subjects No. 127. London: HMSO, 1971.

60.   Committee on the Child Health Services (Chairman, D Court). Fit for the future, Vol. I. Cmnd 6684. London: HMSO, 1976.

61.   Department of Health and Social Security. Priorities for health and personal social services in England. London: HMSO, 1976.

62.   Department of Health and Social Security. The way forward. London: HMSO, 1977.

63.   Social Services Committee (Chairman, R Short). Perinatal and neonatal mortality. Second report from the Social Services Committee, Session 1979-80, Vol. I, HC 663-I. London: HMSO, 1980.

64.   Macfarlane AJ. Variations in numbers of births and perinatal mortality by day of the week. British Medical Journal 1979; 1: 750-751.

65. Maternity Services Advisory Committee. Maternity care in action. Part II. Care during childbirth (intrapartum care); a guide to good practice and a plan for action. London: HMSO, 1984.

66. Campbell R, Macfarlane AJ. Recent debate on the place of birth. In: Garcia J, Kilpatrick R, Richards M, eds. The politics of maternity care. Oxford: Clarendon Press, 1990.

67. Kitzinger S, Davis JA, eds. The place of birth. Oxford: Oxford University Press, 1978.

68. Office of Population Censuses and Surveys. Mortality statistics, perinatal and infant: social and biological factors, England and Wales, Series DH3. London: HMSO, published annually.

69. Glazener CMA, MacArthur GJ. Postnatal care: time for a change. Contemporary Reviews in Obstetrics and Gynaecology 1993; 5:130-136.

70. Garcia J, Kilpatrick R, Richards M, eds. The politics of maternity care. Oxford: Clarendon Press, 1990.

71. Kramer MS. Determinants of low birthweight. Bulletin of the World Health Organisation 1987; 65:663-737.

72. Fryer JG, Ashford A. Trends in perinatal and neonatal mortality in England and Wales 1960-69. British Journal of Preventative and Social Medicine 1972; 26:1-9.

73. Brimblecombe FSW, Ashford JR, Fryer JG. Significance of low birthweight in perinatal mortality. British Journal of Preventative and Social Medicine 1968; 22:27-35.

74. Pethybridge RJ, Ashford JR, Fryer JG. Some features of the distribution of birthweight of human infants. British Journal of Preventative and Social Medicine 1974; 28:10-18.

75. Parsons L, Macfarlane AJ, Golding J. Pregnancy, birth and maternity care. In: Ahmad W, ed. Race and health in contemporary Britain. Milton Keynes: Open University Press, 1993.

76. Chalmers I, Newcombe RG, West RR, et al. Adjusted perinatal mortality rates in administrative areas in England and Wales. Health Trends 1978; 10:24-29.

77. Mallet R, Knox EG. Standardised perinatal mortality ratios: technique, utility and interpretation. Community Medicine 1979; 1:6-13.

78. Macfarlane AJ, Chalmers I, Adelstein AM. The role of standardisation in the interpretation of perinatal mortality rates. Health Trends 1980; 3:45-50.

79. Wilcox AJ, Russell IT. Standardising for birthweight is biased. American Journal of Epidemiology 1983; 18:857-864.

80. Wilcox AJ, Russell IT. Birthweight and perinatal mortality III. Toward a new method of analysis. International Journal of Epidemiology 1986; 15:188-196.

81. Barry CN. Home versus hospital confinement. Journal of the Royal College of General Practitioners 1980; 30:102-107.

82. Zander L. Home v hospital delivery. Journal of Maternal and Child Health 1976; 1:14-20.

83. Curzen P, Mountrose YM. The general practitioner's role in the management of labour. British Medical Journal 1976; 2:1433-1434.

84. Chalmers I. The implications of the current debate on obstetric practice. In: Kitzinger S, Davies JN, eds. The place of birth. Oxford: Oxford University Press, 1978.

85. Shaw B. Preface to 'The doctor's dilemma'. London: Constable and Co., 1906.

86. Enkin MW, Keirse MJNC, Renfrew MJ, et al. Cochrane database of systematic reviews. Pregnancy and childbirth module. Oxford: Update Software, 1993.

87. Lilford RJ. Clinical experimentation in obstetrics. British Medical Journal 1987; 295:1298-1300.

88. Chapman MG, Jones M, Spring JE, et al. The use of a birthroom: a randomized controlled trial comparing delivery with that in the labour ward. British Journal of Obstetrics and Gynaecology 1986; 93:183-187.

89. MacVicar J, Dobbie G, Owen-Johnstone L, et al. Simulated home delivery in hosptial: a randomised controlled trial. British Journal of Obstetrics and Gynaecology 1993; 100:316-323.

90.   Oakley A. Who's afraid of the randomised controlled trial? Some dilemmas of the scientific method and 'good' research practice. In: Roberts H, ed. Women's health counts. London: Routledge, 1990. 167-194.

91.   Klein M, Lloyd I, Redman C, et al. A comparison of a sample of low-risk women delivering in two systems of care - shared care (consultant team) and community care (integrated general practice [GP] unit). Paper presented at 'Pregnancy care for the 1980s' held at the Royal Society of Medicine, 1980.

92.   Elwood JH. Some epidemiological observations on early mortality and birthweight in Belfast. PhD Thesis. The Queen's University, Belfast: Unpublished.

93.   Rose G, Marmot MG. Social class and coronary heart disease. British Heart Journal 1981; 45:13-19.

94.   House of Commons Health Committee. Maternity services. Minutes of evidence, Wednesday July 3 1991. HC 430-v. London: HMSO, 1991.

95.   Chalmers I, Zlosnik JE, Johns KA, Campbell H. Obstetric practice and outcome of pregnancy in Cardiff residents 1965-1973. British Medical Journal 1976; i:735-8.

96.   Barron SL, Thomson AM, Philips PR. Home and hospital confinement in Newcastle upon Tyne 1960-69. British Journal of Obstetrics and Gynaecology 1977; 84:401-11.

97.   Tew M. The case against hospital deliveries: the statistical evidence. In: Kitzinger S, Davis JA, eds. The place of birth. Oxford: Oxford University Press, 1978.

98.   Tew M. Understanding intranatal care through mortality statistics. In: Zander L, Chamberlain G, eds. Pregnancy care for the 1980s. London: Royal Society of Medicine and Macmillan, 1980.

99.   Treffers PE, Laan R. Regional perinatal mortality and regional hospitalisation at delivery in the Netherlands. British Journal of Obstetrics and Gynaecology 1986; 93:690-693.

100.   Ashford JR. Policies for maternity care in England and Wales: too fast and too far? In: Kitzinger S, Davis JA, eds. The place of birth. Oxford: Oxford University Press, 1978.

101. Scherjon S. A comparison between the organisation of obstetrics in Denmark and the Netherlands. British Journal of Obstetrics and Gynaecology 1986; 93:684-689.

102. Savage A. Personal view. British Medical Journal 1981; 283:227.

103. Keirse MJNC. Perinatal mortality rates do not contain what they purport to contain. Lancet 1984; i:1164-1168.

104. Loudon I. On maternal and infant mortality 1900-1960. Social History of Medicine 1991; 4:29-73.

105. Rentoul R. An address: is it in the best interests of public health that the proposed plan of supplying poorer women only with midwives should be opposed and, if so, how are midwives to be done without? Lancet 1897; i:153-159.

106. Local Government Board. Maternal mortality in connection with childbearing. In: Supplement to the forty-fourth annual report of the Local Government Board 1914-15. Cd 8153. London: HMSO, 1916.

107. Campbell J, Cameron ID, Jones DM. High maternal mortality in certain areas. Reports on public health and medical subjects No. 68. London: HMSO, 1932.

108. Grant A. Unpublished observations.

109. Kerr JMM, MacLennan HR. An investigation into the mortality in maternity hospitals. Lancet 1932; i:633-637.

110. Ministry of Health. Interim report of Departmental Committee on Maternal Mortality and Morbidity. London: HMSO, 1930.

111. Holland E. Maternal mortality. Lancet 1935; i:973-976.

112. General Register Office. The Registrar General's decennial supplement, England and Wales, 1931. Part IIa. Occupational mortality. London: HMSO, 1938.

113. Ministry of Health. Report on an investigation into maternal mortality. Cmd 5422. London: HMSO, 1937.

114. Loudon I. Puerperal fever, the streptococcus and sulphonamides 1911-1945. British Medical Journal 1987; 295:485-90.

115.   Ministry of Health. Report on confidential enquiries into maternal deaths in England and Wales 1952-54. Reports on public health and medical subjects No. 97. London: HMSO, 1957.

116.   Ministry of Health. Report on confidential enquiries into maternal deaths in England and Wales 1955-57. Reports on public health and medical subjects No. 103. London: HMSO, 1960.

117.   Ministry of Health. Report on confidential enquiries into maternal deaths in England and Wales 1958-60. Reports on public health and medical subjects No. 108. London: HMSO, 1963.

118.   Department of Health and Social Security. Report on confidential enquiries into maternal deaths in England and Wales 1979-81. Reports on health and social subjects No. 29. London: HMSO, 1986.

119.   Department of Health and Social Security. Report on confidential enquiries into maternal deaths in England and Wales 1982-84. Reports on health and social subjects No. 34. London: HMSO, 1989.

120.   Department of Health, Welsh Office, Northern Ireland Office, Scottish Home and Health Department, Department of Health and Social Services Northern Ireland. Report on confidential enquiries into maternal deaths in the United Kingdom 1985-87. London: HMSO, 1991.

121.   Ministry of Health. The selection of maternity cases for admission to hospital. London: Ministry of Health, 1951.

122.   Morris JN, Heady JA. Social and biological factors in infant mortality I. Objects and methods. Lancet 1955; i:343-349.

123.   Heady JA, Daly C, Morris JN. Social and biological factors in infant mortality II. Variation of mortality with mother's age and parity. Lancet 1955; ii:395-397.

124.   Ministry of Health. Chief Medical Officer's report for 1955. London: HMSO, 1956.

125.   Heady JA, Morris JN. Social and biological factors in infant mortality VI. Mothers who have their babies in hospitals and nursing homes. British Journal of Preventive and Social Medicine 1956; 10:97-106.

126.   Ministry of Health. Chief Medical Officer's report for 1956. London: HMSO, 1957.

127.   Butler NR, Alberman ED. Perinatal problems. The second report of the British Perinatal Mortality Survey. Edinburgh and London: Livingstone, 1969.

128.   Cookson I. Family-doctor obstetrics. Lancet 1963; ii:1051-1054.

129.   Hobbs MST, Acheson ED. Obstetric care in the first pregnancy. Lancet 1966; i:761-764.

130.   Hudson CK. Domiciliary obstetrics in a group practice. Practitioner 1968; 201:816-822.

131.   House of Commons. Official report Session 1984-85. Reply to a written question by John Patten. Hansard. (Parliamentary debates) 70:878-884.

132.   Reynolds JL, Yudkin PL, Bull MJV. General practitioner obstetrics: does risk prediction work? Journal of the Royal College of General Practitioners 1988; 38:307-310.

133.   Bakketeig LS, Hoffman HJ. Perinatal mortality by birth order within cohorts based on sibship size. British Medical Journal 1979; 2:693-696.

134.   Department of Health, Office of Population Censuses and Surveys. Hospital in-patient enquiry maternity tables, 1982-85, England, Series MB4 no 28. London: HMSO, 1988.

135.   House of Commons. Written reply 10 June. Hansard. (Official report) 1991; 192:col 446.

136.   Macfarlane AJ, Campbell R. A review of risks which would be associated with the decision to admit selected primiparous women to the midwifery unit at the Royal Bournemouth General Hospital. Paper prepared for Wessex Regional Health Authority, December 1991.

137.   Van Alten D, Eskes M, Treffers P. Midwifery in the Netherlands. The Wormeveer study; selection, mode of delivery, perinatal mortality and infant morbidity. British Journal of Obstetrics and Gynaecology 1989; 96:656-662.

138.   Ashley J. Personal communication.

139. Richards ID, Donald EM, Hamilton FMW. Use of maternity care in Glasgow. In: McLachan G, Shegog R, eds. In the beginning: studies of maternity services. London: Nuffield Provincial Hospitals Trust, 1970.

140. Chamberlain R, Chamberlain G, Hewlett B, et al. British births 1970, volume I. The first week of life. London: Heinemann, 1975.

141. Klein M, Lloyd I, Redman C, et al. A comparison of low risk pregnant women booked for delivery in two systems of care. British Journal of Obstetrics and Gynaecology 1983; 90:118-122.

142. Tew M. Place of birth and perinatal mortality. Journal of the Royal College of General Practitioners 1985; 35:390-394.

143. Senn SJ. Unpublished analyses.

144. Murphy JF, Dauncey M, Gray OP, et al. Planned and unplanned deliveries at home: implications of a changing ratio. British Medical Journal 1984; 288:1429-1432.

145. Tew M. Changing childbirth. London: Chapman and Hall, 1990.

146. Tew M. The safest place of birth. Lancet 1979; i:1388-1390.

147. Senn SJ. Letter. Lancet 1979; ii:523.

148. Tew M. Letter. Lancet 1979; ii:523-524.

149. Newcombe RG. A statistical view of risk factors. In: Marsh GN, ed. Modern obstetrics in general practice. Oxford: Oxford University Press, 1985.

150. Campbell R, Macdonald Davies I, Macfarlane AJ, et al. Home births in England and Wales; perinatal mortality according to intended place of delivery. British Medical Journal 1984; 289: 721-724.

151. Tew M. Effects of scientific obstetrics on perinatal mortality. Health Services Journal 1981; 91:444-446.

152. Campbell R, Macdonald Davies I, Macfarlane AJ. Perinatal mortality and place of delivery. Population Trends 1982; 28:9-12.

153.   Gunn P. Home deliveries. In: Chamberlain G Gunn, P, eds. Birthplace. Report of the confidential enquiry into facilities available at the place of birth. Chichester: John Wiley, 1987.

154.   Wood LAC. Obstetric retrospect. Journal of the Royal College of General Practitioners 1981; 31:80-90.

155.   Fedrick J, Butler NR. Intended place of delivery and perinatal outcome. British Medical Journal 1978; i:763-765.

156.   Tew M. Intended place of delivery and perinatal outcome. Letter. British Medical Journal 1978; i:1139-1140.

157.   Tew M. Do obstetric intranatal interventions make birth safer? British Journal of Obstetrics and Gynaecology 1986; 93: 659-674.

158.   Rees HGSM. A domiciliary obstetric practice 1948-1958. Journal of the Royal College of General Practitioners 1961; 4:47-71.

159.   Rutter P. Domiciliary midwifery is it justifiable? Lancet 1964; ii:1228-1230.

160.   Woodall J. No place like home. Proceedings of the Royal Society of Medicine 1968; 61:1032-1034.

161.   Tew M. Safety in intranatal care - the statistics. In: Marsh G, ed. Modern obstetrics in general practice. Oxford: Oxford University Press, 1985.

162.   Richmond GA. An analysis of 3,199 patients booked for delivery in general practitioner obstetric units. Journal of the Royal College of General Practitioners 1977; 27:406-413.

163.   Taylor GW, Edgar W, Taylor BA, et al. How safe is general practitioner obstetrics? Lancet 1980; ii:1287-1289.

164.   Lloyd G. Retrospective normality: a comparison of the outcome of pregnancy of women booked in a GP maternity unit and a GP obstetric unit. Practitioner 1975; 214:261-263.

165.   Owen JD. A review of the general practitioner obstetric service in Colchester. Journal of the Royal College of General Practitioners 1981; 31:92-96.

166.   Golding J, Peters T. Are hospital confinements really bad for the
        fetus? Early Human Development 1988; 17:29-36.

167.   Clarke M, Mason ES, MacVicar J, et al. Evaluating perinatal mortality
        rates: effects of referral and case mix. British Medical Journal 1993;
        306:824-7.

168.   Cole SK, Macfarlane AJ. Safety and place of delivery in Scotland.
        Journal of Public Health Medicine. Accepted for publication.

169.   Steering Group on Health Services Information. Supplement to the
        first and fourth reports to the Secretary of State. London: HMSO,
        1985.

170.   House of Commons. Written parliamentary reply. Hansard 1994; July
        18:col 11-12.

171.   McGregor RM, Martin LVH. Obstetrics in general practice. Journal of
        the Royal College of General Practitioners 1961; 4: 542-551.

172.   Banwell GS, Hamilton IG. Use of maternity beds in a new general
        practitioner unit. Journal of the Royal College of General Practitioners
        1970; 19:282-5.

173.   Oldershaw KL, Brudenell JM. Use by general practitioners of obstetric
        beds in a consultant unit: a further report. British Medical Journal
        1975; 1:139-142.

174.   James DK. Patients transferred in labour from general practitioner
        maternity units. Journal of the Royal College of General Practitioners
        1977; 27:414-418.

175.   Lowe SW, House W, Garrett T. Comparison of outcome of low- risk
        labour in an isolated general practice maternity unit and a specialist
        maternity hospital. Journal of the Royal College of General
        Practitioners 1987; 37:484-7.

176.   Garret T, House W, Lowe SW. Outcome of women booked into an
        isolated general practitioner maternity unit over eight years. Journal of
        the Royal College of General Practitioners 1987; 37: 488-90.

177.   Marsh GN, Channing DM. Audit of 26 years of obstetrics in general
        practice. British Medical Journal 1989; 298:1077-80.

178.   Ford C, Illiffe S, Franklin O. Outcome of planned home births in an inner city practice. British Medical Journal 1991; 303:1517-1519.

179.   Smith LFP, Jewell D. Contribution of general practitioners to hospital intrapartum care in maternity units in England and Wales in 1988. British Medical Journal 1991; 302:13-16.

180.   Campbell R, Macfarlane AJ, Cavenagh S. Choice and chance in low risk maternity care. British Medical Journal 1991; 303:1487-88.

181.   Littlepage BNC. General practitioner maternity units. Journal of the Royal College of General Practitioners 1976; 26:263-265.

182.   Young G. Are isolated maternity units run by general practitioners dangerous? British Medical Journal 1987; 294:744-746.

183.   Street P, Gannon MJ, Holt EM. Community obstetric care in West Berkshire. British Medical Journal 1991; 302:698-700.

184.   Wiltshire Healthcare Trust. Unpublished data.

185.   Campbell R. The place of birth. In: Alexander J, Levy V, Roch S, eds. Intrapartum care. A research based approach. Basingstoke: Macmillan, 1990.

186.   Cavenagh AJM, Phillips KM, Sheridan B, Williams EMJ. Contributions of isolated general practitioner maternity units. British Medical Journal 1984; 288:1438-40.

187.   Leader. What future for small obstetric units? Lancet 1985; 2:423-424.

188.   Martin J. Red house mothers renew their fight. St Albans Review 1984; March 22nd.

189.   Warshal S. How to oppose a GP unit closure. Association for Improvements in the Maternity Services.

190.   National Childbirth Trust. Small units resource list. London: NCT, 1993.

191.   Jewell D. General practitioner obstetrics. Time to think again about GP deliveries. British Medical Journal 1989; 298:690-696.

192.   Marsh GN, Cashman HA, Russell IT. General practitioner obstetrics in the Northern Region in 1983. British Medical Journal 1985; 290:901-903.

193.   Prentice A, Walton SM. Outcome of pregnancies referred to a general practitioner maternity unit in a district hospital. British Medical Journal 1989; 299:1090-2.

194.   Bryce FC, Clayton JK, Randf RJ, et al. General practitioner obstetrics in Bradford. British Medical Journal 1990; 300:725-7.

195.   Smith LP. General practice obstetrics in Bradford. Letter. British Medical Journal 1990; 300:875.

196.   Bahrami J, Haywood K, Givans RJ. General practice obstetrics in Bradford. Letter. British Medical Journal 1990; 300:873.

197.   Young GL. General practice obstetrics in Bradford. Letter. British Medical Journal 1990; 300:874.

198.   Ross M, Brooke M, Connolly J, et al. General practice obstetrics in Bradford. Letter. British Medical Journal 1990; 300:1139-40.

199.   Rhodes J, Tedd CB, Roberts HE, et al. General practice obstetrics in Bradford. Letter. British Medical Journal 1990; 300:1140-41.

200.   Mugford M. Unpublished observations.

201.   Black N. Do general practitioner deliveries constitute a perinatal mortality risk? British Medical Journal 1982; 284:488-90.

202.   Sangala V, Dunster G, Bohin S, et al. Perinatal mortality rates in isolated general practitioner maternity units. British Medical Journal 1990; 301:418-20.

203.   Campbell R, Macfarlane AJ. General practitioner maternity units. Letter. British Medical Journal 1990; 301:983-4.

204.   Young GL. General practitioner maternity units. Letter. British Medical Journal 1990; 301:665-6.

205.   Charney M. General practitioner maternity units. Letter. British Medical Journal 1990; 301:664-5.

206.   Zander L, Klein M. Role of the family practitioner in maternity care. In: Chalmers I, Enkin M, Kierse MJNC, eds. Effective care in pregnancy and childbirth. Oxford: Oxford University Press, 1989.

207.   House of Commons. Written reply 5 November. Hansard. (Official report) 1991; 198:col 102.

208.   Richardson A. Personal communication.

209.   Garcia J. Personal communication.

210.   Social Services Committee. Perinatal and neonatal mortality: follow-up. Third report from the Social Services Committee Session 1983-84. HC308. London: HMSO, 1984.

211.   Chamberlain GVP, Gunn P, eds. Birthplace. Chichester: National Birthday Trust Fund & John Wiley and Sons, 1987.

212.   Rosenblatt RA, Deinken J, Shoemack P. Is obstetrics safe in small hospitals? Evidence from New Zealand's regionalised perinatal system. Lancet 1985; 2:429-431.

213.   Lumley J. The safety of small maternity hospitals in Victoria 1982-84. Community Health Studies 1988; xii:386-93.

214.   Hemminki E. Perinatal mortality distributed by type of hospital in the central district of Helskinki, Finland. Scandinavian Journal of Social Medicine 1985; 13:113-118.

215.   Matthews AEB, Shearman WH, Steffens EM. The West Middlesex Hospital Community Obstetric Project. Health Trends 1975; 7:69-71.

216.   Ministry of Health. Annual report of the Chief Medical Officer for 1963. London: HMSO, 1964.

217.   Rawlings EE. A general practitioner short-stay delivery unit. Practitioner 1970; 204:825-830.

218.   Flint C, Poulengeris P, Grant A. The Know Your Midwife scheme - a randomised trial of continuity of care by a team of midwives. Midwifery 1989; 5:11-16.

219.   Allison J. Midwives step out of the shadows. Sir William Power Memorial Lecture. Midwives Chronicle 1992; 105:167-174.

220. Simms C, McHaffie H, Renfrew MJ, Ashurst H, eds. The Midwifery Research Database MIRIAD. A sourcebook of information about research in midwifery. Hale: Books for Midwives Press, 1994.

221. Maitland F. Personal communication.

222. Dawson J. Personal communication.

223. MacVicar J. Personal Communication.

224. Towler J, Bramall J. The midwife in history and society. London: Croom Helm, 1986.

225. Weig M. Audit of independent midwifery 1980-1991. London: Royal College of Midwives, 1993.

226. Chamberlain G, Philipp E, Hewlett B, et al. British births 1970, volume 2. Obstetric care. London: Heinemann, 1978.

227. Jarvis SN, Holloway JS, Hey E. Increase in cerebral palsy in normal birthweight babies. Archives of Disease in Childhood 1985; 60:1113-21.

228. Damstra-Wijmenga SMI. Home confinement: the positive results in Holland. Journal of the Royal College of General Practitioners 1984; 34:425-30.

229. Alment EAJ, Barr A, Reid M, et al. Normal confinement: a domiciliary and hospital study. British Medical Journal 1967; 2: 530-35.

230. Dixon EA. Review of maternity patients suitable for home delivery. British Medical Journal 1982; 284:1753-1755.

231. Klein M, Elbourne D, Lloyd I. Booking for maternity care, a comparison of two systems. Occasional paper 31. London: Royal College of General Practitioners, 1985.

232. Shearer JML. Five year prospective survey of risk of booking for a home birth. British Medical Journal 1985; 291:1478-80.

233. Mehl LE. The outcome of home delivery: research in the United States. In: Kitzinger S, Davis JA, eds. The place of birth. Oxford: Oxford University Press, 1978.

234. House of Commons. Written reply by Mr Sackville. Hansard. (Parliamentary debates) 1992; June 19:col 706.

235.   Mugford M. Economies of scale and low risk maternity care: what is the evidence? Maternity Action 1990; 46:6-8.

236.   Ferster G, Pethybridge R. The cost of a local maternity care system. Hospital and Health Services Review 1973; July:243-247.

237.   Gray AM, Steele R. The economics of specialist and general practitioner maternity units. Journal of the Royal College of General Practitioners 1981; 31:586-592.

238.   Stilwell JA. Relative costs of home and hospital confinements. British Medical Journal 1979; 2:257-9.

239.   Soper J, Jones J. Cost-effectiveness of surgery in small acute 'local' hospitals. Community Medicine 1985; 7:257-264.

240.   Scottish Office Home and Health Department. Provision of maternity services in Scotland. A policy review. Edinburgh: HMSO, 1993.

241.   Department of Health. Changing childbirth. Part I. Report of the Expert Maternity Group. London: HMSO, 1993.

242.   Gordon I, Elias Jones TF. The place of confinement: home or hospital? The mother's preference. British Medical Journal 1960; 1:52-3.

243.   Goldthorp WO, Richman J. Maternal attitudes to unintended home confinement. A case study of the effects of the hospital strike upon domiciliary confinements. Practitioner 1974; 212:845-53.

244.   Fluery PM. Maternity care. Mothers' experience of childbirth. London: Allen and Unwin, 1967.

245.   Campbell R. A study of selected aspects of the change in the place of confinement with particular reference to Plymouth. School of Environmental Sciences, Plymouth Polytechnic: 1979. Unpublished.

246.   O'Brien M. Home and hospital confinement: a comparison of the experiences of mothers having home and hospital confinements. Journal of the Royal College of General Practitioners 1978; 28: 460-6.

247.   Leader. Medicine on television. British Medical Journal 1975; 1:539.

248.   Leader. Induction of labour. British Medical Journal 1976; 1:729-30.

249. Leader. A place to be born. British Medical Journal 1976; 1:55-56.

250. Gillie O. Hospital v home childbirth row looms. Sunday Times 1980; 16 November:6.

251. Loudon I. Obstetrics and the general practitioner. British Medical Journal 1990; 301:703-707.

252. Martin C. How do you count maternal satisfaction? A user commissioned survey of maternity services. In: Roberts H, ed. Women's health counts. London: Routledge, 1990.

253. Cartwright A. The dignity of labour. A study of childbearing and induction. London: Tavistock, 1979.

254. Sheppardson B. Home or hospital births? A study of women's attitudes. Health Visitor 1983; 56:405-406

255. Caplan M, Madeley RJ. Home deliveries in Nottingham 1980-81. Public Health 1985; 99:307-13.

256. Kitzinger S. Women's experiences of birth at home. In: Kitzinger S, Davis JA, eds. The place of birth. Oxford: Oxford University Press, 1978.

257. Jacoby A, Cartwright A. Finding out about the views and experiences of maternity service users. In: Garcia J, Kilpatrick R and Richards M, eds. The politics of maternity care. Oxford: Oxford University Press, 1990.

258. Morgan BM, Bulpitt C, Clifton P, et al. The consumers' attitude to obstetric care. British Journal of Obstetrics and Gynaecology 1984; 91:624-8.

259. Johnson M, Smith J, Haddad S, Walker J, Wong A. Women prefer hospital births. Letter. British Medical Journal 1992; 305:255.

260. Zander L, Chamberlain G, eds. Pregnancy care for the 1980s. London: Royal Society of Medicine and Macmillan, 1983.

261. Campbell R, Macfarlane AJ. Place of delivery: a review. British Journal of Obstetrics and Gynaecology 1986; 93:675-683.

262. Alberman E. Commentary. The place of birth. British Journal of Obstetrics and Gynaecology 1986; 93:657-658.

263. Alberman E. Evidence given to House of Commons Health Committee. In: House of Commons Health Committee. Maternity services. Vol II, Minutes of evidence. HC 29-II. London: HMSO, 1992.

264. House of Commons. Written reply by Mrs Currie. Hansard (Parliamentary debates) 1987; Nov 6:col 919.

265. House of Commons. Written reply by Mr Mellor. Hansard. (Parliamentary debates) 1989; March 21:col 572.

266. House of Commons. Written reply. Hansard. (Parliamentary debates) 1990; July 19:col 705.

267. Royal College of Obstetricians and Gynaecologists. Report of the RCOG Working Party on Antenatal and Intrapartum care. London: RCOG, 1982.

268. Joint Working Party of the Association of Anaesthetists, Obstetric Anaesthetists Association. Anaesthetic services in obstetrics - plan for the future. London: Association of Anaesthetists, 1988.

269. Health Visitors' Association, Royal College of Midwives. Joint statement on the post-natal period. London: HVA and RCM, 1983.

270. Royal College of Midwives. Towards a healthy nation. London: RCM, 1987.

271. President of The Royal College of Obstetricians and Gynaecologists, President of the Royal College of Midwives, President of the Royal College of General Practitioners. Maternity care in the new NHS. A joint approach. London: RCOG, RCM, RCGP, 1992.

272. Bottomley V. Oral evidence given to the House of Commons Health Committee on February 16 1991. In: House of Commons Health Committee. Maternity Services. Vol II, Minutes of evidence. HC 29-II. London: HMSO, 1992.

273. Bottomley V. Oral evidence given to the House of Commons Health Committee on November 11 1991. In: House of Commons Health Committee. Maternity services. Vol II, Minutes of evidence. HC 29-II. London: HMSO, 1992.

274. House of Commons Health Committee, (Chairman N Winterton). Maternity services. Vol I, report. HC 29-I. London: HMSO, 1992.

275. Hunt L. MPs want more women to give birth at home. Independent 1992; March 5:1.

276. Mihill C. MPs back more home births with midwives in charge. Guardian 1992; March 5.

277. Royal College of Obstetricians and Gynaecologists. Complete response to the report of the House of Commons Health Committee on maternity services. London: RCOG, 1992.

278. Department of Health. Maternity services. The Government's response to the second report from the Health Committee, Session 1991-92, Cm 2018. London: HMSO, 1992.

279. Ritchie OH, Dick D, Lingham R. The report of the inquiry into the care and treatment of Christopher Clunis. London: HMSO, 1994.

280. Maternity Unit Study Team. A study of midwife and GP led maternity units. London: Department of Health, 1993.

281. Women to be given control over births. Independent 1993; August 8.

282. Danger seen in backing for home births. Guardian 1993; August 8.

283. Royal College of Midwives. Implementing changing childbirth. The response of the Royal College of Midwives. London: Royal College of Midwives, 1993.

284. Royal College of General Practitioners. Comments on the Expert Maternity Group's report "Changing childbirth". London: Royal College of General Practitioners, 1993.

285. Consultants condemn birth report as cash-saving ploy. BMA News Review 1993; September:10.

286. Royal College of Obstetricians. Press release. August 6 1993.

287. Royal College of Obstetricians and Gynaecologists. Response to the report of the Expert Maternity Group "Changing childbirth". London: RCOG, 1993.

288. Chamberlain G. Birth at home. London: Royal College of Obstetricians and Gynaecologists, 1994.

289.   Welsh Health Planning Forum. Protocol for investment in health gain: maternal and early child health. Cardiff: NHS Directorate, 1992.

290.   Department of Health. Women will have a greater say in maternity care: mother and baby come first. Press release 94/34. January 24 1994. London: Department of Health.

291.   NHS Management Executive. Woman-centred maternity services. Executive letter EL(94)9, January 24 1994.

292.   Department of Health. Baroness Cumberlege announces membership of Advisory Group on 'Changing childbirth'. Press release 94/225. London: Department of Health May 10 1994.

293.   NHS. The patient's charter. Maternity services. Leeds: Department of Health, 1994.

294.   Department of Health. Greater choice for women in maternity services. Press release 94/200. London: Department of Health, April 22 1994.

295.   Department of Health, Welsh Office, Northern Ireland Office, Scottish Home and Health Department, Department of Health and Social Services Northern Ireland. Report on confidential enquiries into maternal deaths in the United Kingdom 1988-90. London: HMSO, 1994.

296.   Streetly A. Maternity care in the 90s. Health For All 2000 News 1994; 26:14-15.

297.   Maternity Alliance. Born in poverty. Maternity Action 1993; 61:9.

298.   Campbell R, Macfarlane AJ. Obstetrics and the general practitioner. Letter. British Medical Journal 1990; 301:1103.

299.   Commission for Racial Equality. Race relations code of practice in maternity services. London: CRE, 1994.

Index